Psychotherapy Case Studies

Psychotherapy Case Studies is composed of 11 compelling and emotionally intimate stories that illuminate the hidden psychological forces shaping our lives and the path to genuine freedom. These jargon-free narratives re-envision therapy as a sacred journey in which the therapist accompanies patients through their deepest struggles and creates an accepting home for the full spectrum of their lives.

Through stories spanning the depths of psychological despair and the heights of spiritual illumination, the book weaves Eastern contemplative and Western psychoanalytic wisdom, demonstrating the extraordinary healing that is possible when the therapist is like an emotional jazz improviser who is free and creative and approaches each person as unique. Each case reveals our unsuspected capacity not just to cope, but to thrive amid life's challenges.

Written for both beginning and seasoned therapists, students of psychology, and anyone curious about the transformative power of authentic human connection, these inspiring stories offer sustenance and hope in challenging times.

Jeffrey B. Rubin, PhD, is a psychoanalytically oriented therapist in New York and a Sensei in the Nyogen Senzaki and Soen Nakagawa Zen tradition. He is the author of six books on the integration of Eastern and Western approaches to flourishing and self-transformation. Rubin has taught at various psychoanalytic institutes and meditation, yoga and growth centers around the country and abroad including the United Nations, Union Theological Seminary, the Esalen Institute, and the 92nd Street Y. His pioneering approach to therapy was featured in the *New York Times* magazine.

"In this masterfully crafted work, Jeffrey B. Rubin weaves together the wisdom of Eastern contemplative traditions with the depth of psychoanalytic understanding through the timeless power of storytelling. His compelling narratives—spanning from sports fields to Zen temples, from clinical breakthroughs to therapeutic failures—reimagine the therapeutic relationship as a sacred encounter, where the therapist, like Virgil guiding Dante, accompanies patients through their deepest struggles. The author's emphasis on the art of deep listening and presence illuminates a path toward authentic healing that is both deeply practical and profoundly transformative. Each story serves as a window into human experience, demonstrating how the artful integration of mindful presence and psychological insight can facilitate genuine transformation. An essential read for clinicians seeking to expand their therapeutic repertoire and for anyone interested in the art of human understanding."

Inna Rozentsvit, MD, PhD, *psychoanalytically trained neurologist, neurorehabilitation and neurodiversity specialist, psychohistorian, publisher, and transdisciplinary researcher*

"Both clinical, philosophical, spiritual, and autobiographical, Jeffrey Rubin's *Psychotherapy Case Studies: Escaping the Prison You Didn't Know You Were In* is a compelling read and an extraordinarily insightful and inspiring self-portrait and account of the work of a truly gifted psychotherapist and thinker. With humor and profound empathy for his patients, Rubin shares his hard-won wisdom with us all, interweaving his life and therapeutic experience, literary and his Zen Buddhist relational intersubjective psychoanalytic perspective, into a wonderful narrative. I highly recommend it for therapists young and old, patients, truth-seekers and anyone who would like a searching, eloquent, and honest look into how psychotherapy really works."

Kenneth Rasmussen, PsyD, PhD, *International Psychohistorical Association, psychotherapist in private practice*

"Through the lens of psychotherapy, Dr. Rubin's book deeply delves into a diverse array of stories, ranging from sports to spirituality, revealing the profound human capacity for resilience and meaning making amidst trauma. Each account offers a powerful reminder that, while we may feel overwhelmed, it is possible, even necessary, to confront our fears with clarity and dignity. The emphasis on compassion and understanding in therapy is particularly striking; he advocates for a tender, individualized approach that honors each person's emotional journey, rather than resorting to generic solutions.

The personal experiences shared by the author deepen the impact of the text. The losses endured, including the passing of close family members and friends, serve as a backdrop to the exploration of transformation. This period of grief and introspection not only shaped the author's clinical work but also underscored the importance of connection and hope in a fractured world. This book offers readers both inspiration and guidance. By telling these stories, Dr. Rubin is taking care of the hearts that seek connection."

Joanne Cacciatore, PhD, *Professor at Arizona State University;*
author of Bearing the Unbearable: Love, loss, and the
heartbreaking path of grief

"Jeffrey Rubin's new book, *Psychotherapy Case Studies: Escaping The Prison You Didn't Know You Were In*, is a courageous undertaking, providing a portrait not only of patient dynamics but of Rubin's own defining struggles with himself as he navigates his way through his work with the people he sees in treatment. His approach is a tacit acknowledgment that no meaningful evaluation of psychoanalytic work can unfold without consideration of the intricacies of the therapist's own personality. It is written in a wonderfully clear, lucid, down-to-earth prose that renders consideration of complex case material an easy, enjoyable read. His conception of his therapeutic work is deeply persuasive and insightful. The people whose lives he has chosen to discuss are drawn in vivid, poignant terms. He integrates traditional psychoanalytic concepts with core concepts that define Eastern philosophical approaches, both of which inform his relationship with himself and his orientation to psychotherapy and analysis. As this integration implies, his approach, in a sense, is a non-traditional one: psychotherapy is viewed as an organic endeavor in which concerns about humanity and engagement supersede focus upon prescriptive rules."

Richard Wood, PhD, *Clinical psychology in 1974 (Wayne State University), Founder and Director of the Thornhill Multidisciplinary Assessment Center, Founding member of the Canadian Association of Psychologists in Disability Assessment, and Former President of the Ontario Psychological Association in 1989. He has written three books*

Psychotherapy Case Studies

Escaping the Prison You Didn't Know You Were In

Jeffrey B. Rubin

Routledge
Taylor & Francis Group
LONDON AND NEW YORK

Designed cover image: © Jeffrey B. Rubin

First published 2026
by Routledge
4 Park Square, Milton Park, Abingdon, Oxon OX14 4RN

and by Routledge
605 Third Avenue, New York, NY 10158

Routledge is an imprint of the Taylor & Francis Group, an informa
business

British Library Cataloguing-in-Publication Data
A catalogue record for this book is available from the British Library

ISBN: 978-1-032-99541-0 (hbk)
ISBN: 978-1-032-98724-8 (pbk)
ISBN: 978-1-003-60473-0 (ebk)

DOI: 10.4324/9781003604730

Typeset in Optima
by Apex CoVantage, LLC

This book is dedicated to George Atwood, whose empathy, wisdom, and compassion has been of inestimable importance in my efforts to understand myself and aid suffering souls. Dante never had a better Virgil.

Contents

Acknowledgments

I owe a debt of gratitude to my patients for providing the opportunity to accompany them in their individual journeys and enter their unique worlds. This book—and my life—have been immeasurably enriched by our mutual attempts to investigate and understand their hopes and fears, dreams and conflicts.

Writers don't create in isolation. I am blessed to have friends and colleagues who talked through ideas, read chapters—or the whole manuscript—and provided emotional support and vital feedback. Conversations with Diana Alstad, Nicole D'Andria, George Atwood, Mark Banschick, Aileen Blitz, Joanne Cacciatore, Josh Cohen, Rick DeBenedetto, Paul Elovitz, Mark Finn, Jerry Garguilo, Skye Goldberg, Audrey Jacobson, Sifu Jeff Jones, David Kastan, Peter Knobler, Jesse Kornbluth, Joel Kramer, Alexandra Krithades, Henry Lothane, Ellen Luborsky, John Moody, Lou Mitsunen Nordstrom, Alice Peck, Ken Rasmussen, Inna Rozentsvit, Victor Sahn, Lou Salvucci, Tony Stern, Ann Ulanov, Monte Ullman, Marc Wayne, Leslie Wolowitz, and Richard Wood enriched this manuscript.

I am deeply grateful for the invaluable assistance of George Atwood, Alice Peck, Ken Rasmussen, and Inna Rozentsvit, who ensured that the manuscript crossed the finish line.

Kate Hawes, Deepika Batra, Hannah Rayner, Lauren Ellis, and Jo Hardern from Routledge have been a pleasure to work with every step of the publication process. Jo Steer and Duane Stapp did a stellar job on the cover. Martin Pettitt skillfully edited the manuscript and was a joy to work with.

Permissions

1. Reprinted with permission from the American Psychoanalytic Association. Originally published in *The American Psychoanalyst* (Spring/Summer 2017, Volume 51, No. 2).
2. Rubin, Jeffrey, (2007), From Nowhere to Now-here. In Into the Mountain Stream: Psychotherapy and Buddhist Experience. Ed.: Paul Cooper, Ph.D. (2007 Lanham, MD. Jason Aronson).

Author's Note

This book is a work of nonfiction; however, in order to protect the privacy of individuals, names and identifying details have been changed. The experiences, emotions, and themes explored in these pages are authentic and reflect real encounters, although certain details may have been modified to respect confidentiality.

Preface

"As long as people breathe, they will speak, they will write, and they will tell stories," wrote author Fang Fang (2022) in *Wuhan Diary: Dispatches from a Quarantined City*. Stories are the lifeblood of existence—they are a unique human gift and central to our survival. They help us make sense of the complexity and chaos of experience. They provide guidance and direction. They can bring out the best within.

In a time that is increasingly baffling and heartless, we feel lost and scared, unprotected and powerless. Bedeviled by feelings we do not understand—and were never trained to manage—it is tempting to gravitate toward unsustainable, quick-fix solutions, fundamentalisms, and orthodoxies on both sides of the polarizing spectrum, or retreat into private, insular realms of comfort and solace.

What we hunger for are ways to explain what plagues us. We also yearn to be nourished and inspired. The narratives in this book of people in psychotherapy cover a wide landscape—from sports and spirituality to the creativity in madness and the human capacity to endure and find meaning in the face of emotional devastation and trauma. They teach us it is possible to live with clarity and dignity in times of insanity, bear the unbearable, and not flee from—and attempt to understand—what we fear and detest.

These stories of traumatized children and demoralized couples, suicidal teenagers and alienated Zen masters demonstrate the extraordinary transformation and healing that is possible when we honor people's emotional experience and investigate with patience and empathy the psychological adversity they have undergone, instead of relying on paint-by-numbers approaches in which the person in therapy is subordinated to a one-size-fits-all framework. They shed light on what we are grappling with as we face an uncertain world and embolden us in disturbing times.

I experienced this personally over the past few years, and it greatly enriched my clinical work. My younger brother and I buried our father on Halloween in 2016. Our mother died 11 days later. Then, I lost eight people—friends, relatives (my brother, uncle, and cousin), as well as mentors—within a year. The losses and grief combined with the isolation and self-reflection triggered by

COVID-19 was unexpectedly constructive: it ripped me open and enlarged my heart. The personal and societal challenges illuminated what really mattered: I reconnected with old friends and teachers, returned to and recommitted to former passions like martial arts, and felt deeply troubled by the heartlessness and insanity in the world. What effortlessly resulted was a fierce aspiration to be a counterforce to the madness, as well as a renewed wish to be an ally to people navigating the chaos, the toughness of their lives, and the crushing loneliness and alienation of our weary world.

This book was one of the concrete results of that period of pain and self-examination. I saw with greater clarity and conviction the importance of stories and experiences of grounded hope as an alternative to paralyzing pessimism or empty optimism. It brought me joy to provide what I yearned for as I mourned the loss of the world I knew, and my hope is to offer this to readers.

References

Fang, Fang. *Wuhan Diary: Dispatches from a Quarantined City*. New York: HarperCollins, 2022.

Introduction

He was tortured from the inside. He didn't understand what he felt. He didn't know who he was. He was unsure of what I wanted him to say. He fidgeted so much that I—the psychotherapist who was supposed to be grounded and calm so that I could help him—grew anxious.

I was sitting across from Joel, a shy, skinny, 16-year-old whose parents had brought him to therapy because he was miserable and had no friends.

Joel squirmed on my black couch, averted his eyes, and began looking around my office. First, he scanned the colorful print on the wall—Wilhelm de Kooning's myriad colors, textures, and shapes—which remind me of the richness and complexity of each human being. Then he glanced at the dream-catcher near the statue of the Buddha on the windowsill, shifted his gaze to a photograph of a stone path in Kyoto, and returned to de Kooning.

Joel spoke in a series of broken sentences, halting as if censoring himself before he completed a thought. Words half-formed, sentences begun and stopped suddenly, all delivered in staccato speech. On the rare occasion his eyes met mine they immediately slid away. "What a jerk I was . . . I can't believe how stupid I am . . . I shouldn't have . . ."

Our sessions were like rollercoaster rides. Emotional intimacy was perilous for him. Brief conversations about parents and girls, religion and writing were interspersed with fear and self-consciousness, self-loathing and withdrawal. One minute he was emotionally present, the next he disappeared. His anguish was palpable.

I was lost from week to week, not sure I was really helping him.

Then, early one Saturday morning, my home phone rang. I answered it.

"Hey, Doctor Rubin! How ya doin'?" Joel asked. His voice was animated and un-self-conscious. No terror. No shame. He sounded excited.

According to the "rules" of my psychoanalytic training, Joel was violating the basic therapeutic framework by calling me at home—a classical overstepping of boundaries. But before I could become uptight because of my attachment to preordained ideas about how therapy should unfold, he launched into an animated discussion about his visit to a Buddhist monastery and his

DOI: 10.4324/9781003604730-1

reading about Buddhism and Christianity. Then, seemingly out of nowhere, the familiar shame overwhelmed him.

"I can't believe I called you," he said. "You probably think I'm an idiot . . . a jerk."

I didn't. I was thinking he was incredibly courageous for overcoming his terror and picking up the phone. Calling me was a breakthrough in our relationship.

"I'm much more thought-less than you," I said out loud.

"Yeah. Right. You're an author and a psychotherapist and a professor and I'm nobody. You're full of it!"

I continued. "You are more thought-full than me. You're filled with all sorts of thoughts and imagine that I am condemning and mocking you. But none of that is going on in my mind. I am just listening to you, appreciating your integrity and courage."

He was stunned silent for a moment. Then he laughed. "It was okay to call you."

Patients are generally discouraged from phoning their therapists at home, and when they do it is usually not about happy news. I had not given Joel my home phone number and this was not a scheduled call. Since he wasn't in crisis, I could have followed the rules and told him we'd resume our conversation during our next session, but instinct encouraged me to try something radically different. Over the years I have learned that sometimes I need to drop or suspend what I "know" about therapy or a patient to create enough space in me and between us for the unexpected to emerge.

This practice made it easier to hear what Joel struggled with: he wanted to be valued; he longed for and dreaded intimacy with other people; and he was terrified of my rejection. His call was his creative attempt to challenge his fears and to relate to himself and to me in a new way. That's what made me think his effort to connect with me was more important than the fact that he had called me at home on a weekend, which, in light of what we both learned from the experience, was inconsequential. Had I let him feel in the slightest way that his behavior was inappropriate, I would have lost him to shame and self-denigration.

After that conversation, our relationship and Joel's view of himself gradually grew. He became less self-conscious and made more eye contact. His unrelenting self-contempt lessened. Negative thoughts still arose that made him believe he was inferior, and there were times when, like the man in the Buddhist fable who jumped when he saw the tiger he had painted on the wall of a cave, Joel was imprisoned by the scary pictures he created in his imagination. But fortunately, our interaction helped him realize he was not despicable, that something more than protective isolation was possible, and that he could be close to someone else and not humiliated and endangered.

As months passed, Joel became more like a whole person than a lost soul. He talked to me about his life, the issues he was struggling with, and what he wanted. He began taking risks and venturing beyond the safe and deadening confines of his isolated world.

The transformation after Joel's momentous phone call spurred me to reflect upon what helped him and the principles underlying my view of therapy and change:

- We have a remarkable capacity to symbolize emotional pain. We are all "artists of the underworld" who have an uncanny ability to unconsciously communicate more than we know about where we are trapped and how we might be freed.
- Listen without an agenda. When we don't know what we'll find, we can find what we don't know.
- Decode unconscious, symbolic meaning.
- There is an incomparable power in human understanding. When we cultivate empathy—perceiving someone from within their frame of reference—we provide an emotional home for their feelings which decreases secret shame and fosters healing.
- There is always an emotional logic beneath even apparently destructive and distressing behavior.
- Our symptoms are our teachers—silent memorials to our unwitnessed pain that we hold onto until they are seen and validated to keep alive the hope that love will be forthcoming—rather than toxic presences that must be denied or eliminated.
- We need to cure the patient of what Masud Khan (1974) called their "practice of self-cure" —the emotional splints that protected them as children and now imprison them as adults.
- The therapist is an emotional jazz improviser whose freedom and creativity facilitates optimal responsiveness.
- One size never fits all. Because everyone is unique, we must individualize the treatment.
- Utilize whatever fosters constructive change and healing in the therapist as well as the patient—including emotional connectedness and insight, action and creativity, meditation and conscious breathing.

I'll elaborate.

Human beings have an amazing superpower: an uncelebrated ability to symbolize even the most complex and troubling psychological states and experiences and point toward their transformation. I once worked with an artist who initiated therapy because of a vague and diffuse sense of emotional pain. He experienced himself as worthless and strange, which he had trouble describing. He believed his parents viewed him as despicable and he felt powerless in their presence. After about a year of therapy he had a memory of sketching, many years before, a dwarf that represented for him, "all he hated of himself condensed into one figure." His body. His feeling of being emotionally weird. His conviction of insignificance. His parents' wholesale condemnation of his being. The drawing and his associations to it revealed an unconscious self-image that had haunted him his entire life, which couldn't be transformed until it was depicted. Once the image and the accompanying feelings of self-loathing and alienation were symbolically communicated, we could confront the nightmare together.

Our remarkable ability to listen is a therapist's second superpower. Meditators know that we all have the capacity to cultivate heightened attentiveness, focus, and clarity. Mindfulness—non-judgmental, present-centered attentiveness—is a wonderful gift.

Psychotherapists realize that one more quality is necessary for optimal listening: translating or decoding the hidden meaning of what we hear. When we combine both—I call it the marriage of mindfulness and meaning—we become immeasurably more attuned. And that helps us see other people and ourselves in a dramatically clearer light and respond to them with greater patience and compassion.

Shame is the specter in almost every therapist's office. When a client racked with humiliation detects that the therapist is judgmental, their mortification deepens, they see the therapist as a representative of every disapproving figure in their past, and they protect themselves by shutting down, fleeing, or attacking the therapist. This usually happens on an unconscious level, and the patient (and sometimes even the therapist) is all too often unaware of it, but it erodes the rapport and undermines the therapeutic process. Certain topics become taboo, off-limits, and missed opportunities for deeper understanding.

"In the beginner's mind there are many possibilities, in the expert's mind there are few," wrote Zen teacher Shunryu Suzuki (1970) in *Zen Mind, Beginner's Mind*. A beginner's mind means that we are open and receptive, listening without preconceptions or an agenda. This provides a glimpse of something quite remarkable—what it might mean for each of us to suspend our egocentricity and get out of the way so that the world and people who inhabit it might each speak to us in their own voices.

A passage from one of the core texts of Taoism, the *Tao Te Ching* (translated here by Stephen Mitchell, 2006), teaches us:

When people see some things as beautiful, other things become ugly.
    When people see some things as good, other things become bad.

When the therapist simply listens to the patient and refrains from labeling, resorting to familiar categories, or making conventional distinctions—healthy and sick, acceptable and unacceptable—the therapeutic atmosphere becomes safer and freer, which makes it easier for people like Joel to feel secure and open up.

Unfortunately, all too many therapists, even well-intentioned ones, "shrink" their patients because they "know" too much beforehand about what is "wrong" with the person, what is "supposed" to happen in therapy, and how to conduct the treatment. The therapist becomes a slave of the system that they have mastered. They operate like a customs official who makes sure the therapeutic rules are unfailingly followed and forbids anything deemed "illegal" (like a patient's weekend phone call to his therapist's home) to be smuggled into the process. The patient is stuffed into a one-size-fits-all box. Whatever they say or do is translated into, and becomes proof of, the therapist's particular theory. Trained for years in human dynamics and diagnosis, the therapist treats the patient as an illustration of a syndrome, or a candidate for a quick fix like Zoloft, rather than a unique and complex person. Failure, a topic we'll discuss in Chapter 6, is almost assured.

The best therapy involves the therapist listening to and learning from clients—who they are and what they need—which can change from session to session. If done well, a patient's life—and as you'll see in this book, sometimes a therapist's—can be radically transformed as harmful patterns are exposed, apparently hopeless situations are reconfigured, and annihilating suffering is reduced. Clients experience a vitality and intimacy that they may otherwise have never known.

Meditative Psychotherapy

Integrating the best features of the meditative and psychotherapeutic traditions—what I call *meditative psychotherapy* (Rubin, 2026)—has helped me practice in this way. Studying both methods in tandem cultivates listening with an innocent mind, one that is relatively free of dogma and conventional judgments. This enables us to have much greater access to our own creative thinking and functioning—our relatively untapped capacity for inventive and unpredictable responses that are liberating—as well as hear other people in profoundly deeper and more authentic ways.

When a therapist listens with an innocent mind, they can approach therapeutic challenges—like those I faced on the phone with Joel—in fresh and unexpected ways and dissolve apparent impasses. We can see an excited Saturday morning phone call from a patient as a spontaneous opportunity for a breakthrough, rather than an intrusion.

Good therapists are like emotional jazz improvisers who are grounded in the fundamentals of human development and the therapeutic process and are capable of springing from them in creative response to the demands of the moment.

This isn't always easy to do. We live in a culture that is phobic about feelings and avoids them in a variety of ways. In the current headlong craze to map the brain, overprescribe medications, or offer cognitive short-cuts or workarounds to emotions we can't handle, the field of mental health has failed people in emotional pain. And that causes us to neglect an important fact: symptoms are our teachers. There is always an emotional logic and wisdom beneath even apparently baffling and unalterable challenges in living, from self-cutting and delusions to depression and despair. I believe one of the reasons certain symptoms are resistant to change is that they serve a vital unconscious function: they keep alive the hope that they will be witnessed and the love and acceptance we yearn for will be forthcoming. If we illuminate what our feelings and suffering are communicating instead of ignoring or muting them, we are capable of unsuspected resilience and extraordinary healing.

When the therapist has a jazz-like freedom, every session is an adventure into the unknown, a special connection and exchange devoted to the uniqueness of each patient and flexible enough to individualize treatment by drawing on whatever is useful.

Beyond Psychotherapy

The stories in this book illustrate how therapist and client can discover liberating truths and new ways of relating that can set them free. They also shed new light on the psychology of everyday life—the creative but flawed strategies we use to attempt to heal ourselves that undermine and sabotage us.

Have you ever wondered why you are often your own worst critic or why you don't change, even when you know what is wrong? Is it ever confusing and disturbing that you fail to do what you know is good for you, or don't live up to your most cherished ideals or exercise too little self-discipline? These behaviors seem, on the surface, to be signs of pathology that are both illogical and self-destructive and must be removed. They cause us to go in circles—a kind of groundhog "daze." But while they do hinder us, they have their own emotional logic, even though it is a convoluted one.

My clinical work over four decades with a wide range of people—Buddhist and yoga teachers, gifted and traumatized children, and oppositional teenagers and jaded couples—has taught me that human beings attempt to cope with an emotionally overwhelming world by engaging in an unconscious process of self-protection that I call emotional self-splinting, a creative and makeshift, but ultimately flawed, attempt to heal ourselves.

A physical splint is a protective covering placed on a physical injury such as a sprained ankle or a broken bone that isolates and protects the injury by immobilizing it. Movement is restricted. The risk of re-injury is reduced. Splints are necessary for healing. After the injury has mended, the splint is removed. If it was never taken off, the muscles would atrophy and become weak and inflexible.

Emotional splints are the child's imperfect attempt at self-cure for the psychological tribulations of childhood. They shield us against further emotional injury and pain and protect fragile parts of ourselves. I am thinking of the child who tries to garner love by being perfect in order to justify his existence, and yet never believes he is "good enough"; or the adolescent who isolates from intimacy to never be hurt again; or the adult who compulsively takes care of other people to the exclusion of herself in an attempt to be loved.

I also have in mind the physically abused or terrorized young girl who learns to squelch her feelings throughout her life so she will never provoke other people who might hurt her again, and the young boy who is humiliated by a macho parent when he cries and can't show any vulnerability when he grows up, even to his spouse, for fear of feeling that same mortification.

These unconscious efforts at emotional damage control were once necessary and even creative solutions for what we were grappling with. They helped us survive, but there are also tragic consequences. Immobilizing an emotional injury protects the vulnerable facets of our personalities but ultimately retards our growth and recovery and leads to a calcification of the self—emotional atrophy and inflexibility—that persists into adulthood.

Emotional splints close us off to new experiences and guarantee that we do not learn from them and grow or change. This explains two crucial and troubling features of human life and development: 1) why it is so difficult for most of us to change and 2) why most people repeat what they hate—victims of abuse, for example, who continually find themselves in similar denigrating relationships.

Unless we leave the psychological cells that formerly protected us, we remain entrapped within portable, invisible psychological prisons that undermine our lives. Part of the art of psychotherapy is healing ourselves of the "illness" created by such efforts at self-cure, so that we can lead more fulfilling lives.

In this book I'll depict moments of insight and awakening, risk and change that I have experienced while practicing psychotherapy. How therapy works and what therapists think is seldom revealed. What is the therapist's experience from the other side of the couch? What do they do and why? And what are they thinking about when they do it?

Therapists rarely write about the unorthodox interventions that are sometimes necessary to foster healing. Most movies and novels present skewed and only partially accurate portraits of mental health professionals and the therapeutic process. Therapists in popular culture usually dispense unnecessary prescriptions, pious morality, and superficial advice. "Yet why not say what happened?" as poet Robert Lowell (1977) recommended in "Epilogue." Focusing on the heart of actual therapy sessions without the bias of popular media or the professional jargon that characterizes much writing on therapy and obscures more than it illuminates, I present an insider's view of how therapy works and what helps people grow and change. In each chapter I'll illuminate the empathy and humility, honesty and playfulness, compassion and humor that are necessary for healing to occur. The stories in the book are true—they actually occurred—but they are inevitably incomplete. There is no such thing as a full account of someone's life. And even if there was, it couldn't be expressed on the written page. In each chapter I have focused on indispensable themes and details, designed to give the reader the essence of what happened, but I have altered certain identifying information and eliminated inessential facets to preserve the privacy of the people I write about. In all cases I have striven to honor the spirit of the person, their lives, struggles, and strengths.

There's one question on everybody's mind: "What's in it for me?"

In a world in which we are living at a frenzied pace and increasingly bombarded by information, much of it trivial and addictive, focusing on the return on investment makes a good deal of sense. Otherwise, we waste a lot of time and miss what might be more crucial and self-enhancing.

What's in this book for you—psychotherapists and clients in psychotherapy, spiritual seekers or lay people interested in personal growth—is greater clarity about the hidden forces that shaped you and the prison you didn't know you were in, and access to a life that is more fully your own.

"Nothing can give so keen a pleasure / As helping each and every one," wrote Bertolt Brecht in Leslie Lendrum's 1976 translation of his poem "The Joy of Giving." He went on to say, "What I possess I cannot treasure / Without a mind to pass it on." My hope is that my view from the other side of the couch will not only illuminate universal dilemmas by shining a new light on them, but open your mind, touch your heart, and enrich your life.

References

Brecht, Bertolt. "The Joy of Giving." In *Poems 1913–1956*, edited by John Willett and Ralph Mannheim. New York: Routledge, 1976.

Khan, Masud R. *The Privacy of the Self: Papers on Psychoanalytic Theory and Technique*. United States: International Universities Press, 1974.

Lao Tzu. *Tao Te Ching*. Translated by Stephen Mitchell. New York: Harper, 2006.

Lowell, Robert. "Epilogue." In *Day by Day*. New York: Farrar, Straus & Giroux, 1977.

Rubin, Jeffrey B. *Meditative Psychotherapy and Psychoanalysis: Pathways to Healing and Transformation*. New York: Routledge, 2025.

Suzuki, Shunryu. *Zen Mind, Beginner's Mind*. New York: Weatherhill, 1970.

1 Nothing But Net

How Basketball Led Me to Buddhism and Psychoanalysis

My path to creating meditative psychotherapy began in an unlikely place: the basketball court. Basketball was my first love. It's what I worshipped; what I was whole-heartedly devoted to. I played and practiced by myself for thousands of hours, intoxicated by the rhythm of the game and the joy of teamwork. When I was 18, basketball rewarded me in an unexpected way—it was my first "Zen" meditation teacher.

The memory, five decades later, remains vivid. February 1971. Riverdale, New York. My team was playing an away game against the Fieldston School, a team we were favored to beat. In order to remain in contention for the league title, we had to win. And winning was, unfortunately, next to godliness in our competitive, myopic, adolescent minds.

It was a close, heart-throbbing, hotly contested, roller-coaster battle. When we scored a basket with ten seconds left, our one-point lead appeared bulletproof. But with six seconds to go, they scored. Suddenly we were down by one point. My teammates looked devastated, shell-shocked.

A great calm descended upon me. Five seconds remained on the clock as I called time out. I can still see the panic on my teammates' faces as we huddled close together, the sweat dripping. They had given up.

I stood next to my coach and put my hand on his shoulder. I asked him to tell my teammates to stay calm and get me the ball. "Spread the floor, move without the ball and let Jeffrey take the last shot," Coach said. "If Jeffrey is double-teamed, be ready for him."

Look at your watch. Count out five seconds. It is over so quickly. I had little time to try to do whatever I was going to do. We took the ball out underneath their basket, 94 feet from our goal. The other team lined up down the court, near our basket. They were playing a box-and-one—four of their players played a zone defense, guarding the specific area they were assigned, and one of them, who was 6′ 2″, shadowed me (I was 5′ 7″) wherever I went. A teammate rolled the ball to me near midcourt—the clock wouldn't start until I touched the ball—approximately 45 feet from the hoop.

I am sure there was noise in the gym, but when I dribbled up the left side of the court, the place was as quiet as a Buddhist monastery. I couldn't hear the

DOI: 10.4324/9781003604730-2

crowd, the squeaking of sneakers or the thumping of the basketball. I was in a cocoon of concentration—alert, focused, undistracted, fully and effortlessly in the present, with no thoughts or emotions. My mind was as quiet as it had ever been—Grand Canyon quiet. And clear like the open sky.

Time seemed to slow down and elongate. I floated up court with no sense of exertion—no pressure, no fear. The hope of victory, the dread of losing, did not exist. My opponent didn't faze me. There wasn't really any opponent. Oh, there was someone guarding me, but he had no impact, because, at that moment, he was like a cardboard cutout of a defender standing between the basket and me. It was just the ball, the basket, and me. And we were one. If maintaining that state of harmony meant giving up everything I owned, I wouldn't have hesitated.

As I approached the top of the key, my defender picked me up. I sensed it was time to shoot. I wrapped my left hand around the middle of the ball, my fingertips touching its seams, my right hand cradling the top right-hand corner the way I had practiced for thousands of solitary hours since the fifth grade until it was grooved into my soul. I squared my shoulders to the basket, bent my knees, and jumped in the air. My opponent leaped toward me. I scanned the basket like an archer measuring the target, then released the ball. My left arm was extended, right through the fingertips, straight and true. The palm of my left hand waved to the rim and then faced downward, the way Nat Holman, Clair Bee, Bill Bradley, and countless coaches and players had recommended before the game went airborne and abandoned the fundamental ground from which it was launched.

Just as I released the ball, the arms of my 6' 2" defender enveloped me and blocked my vision so that I could no longer see the rim. As my feet touched the wooden gym floor, there was a cavernous silence. I looked at the basket and saw the net raise skyward, the way it does when a high-arching shot drops cleanly through the hoop. I looked at the scoreboard and realized that my shot had gone in. A deafening roar broke my spell as our fans mobbed the court.

The locker room was noisy, but I was strangely quiet—unmoved by the dramatic win and my personal heroics. I wasn't numb. And I wasn't indifferent to winning; as a highly competitive teenage athlete, victory was very important to me. Our win did not lose its luster because I was upset by the transience of its sweetness. No, I was unemotional about our comeback because victory paled compared to what I had been graced by.

I remember standing alone in the locker room after my teammates had showered and dressed. I remained completely motionless, replaying the last five seconds of the game: the heightened attentiveness, focus, and clarity; the way time seemed to expand; the absence of thought, pressure, and fear; the ecstasy and serenity more joyous than victory or acclaim.

"There is another world, but it is in this one," the novelist Patrick White wrote in *The Solid Mandala* (1983). While my teammates were celebrating our narrow victory, I was preoccupied with the tantalizing glimpse

I'd had of another dimension of being, in which there is whole-hearted, un-self-conscious engagement and intimacy in the moment.

Before the last five seconds of this game, I would have called my childhood—which was devoid of religious training or spiritual realizations—non-religious. What happened in the Fieldston gym became a defining moment in my life. I knew then that there was a radically different way of encountering myself and relating to the world than I had ever been exposed to. The vice-grip of ambition, competitiveness, and victory—the divinities I had worshipped—was loosened.

She plays the piano best who is not concentrating on her fingers. Zen master Yamada Roshi (2015) was fond of saying that "the practice of Zen is to forget the self in the act of uniting with something." In that state of heightened attentiveness, un-self-consciousness, and intimacy (that meditative arts and martial artists call *mushin*), one responds wholeheartedly without thinking. During that basketball game it became clear to me that surrendering to and flowing with life was no less important than planning and goal-directed behavior.

Sports writers and academics claim that sports provide an opportunity to build character and a laboratory to discover the best within oneself. For me, basketball was both of those things, but it was also, like Buddhism was to the Buddha, a raft to another shore. It wasn't until several years later—after I had done intensive meditation practice during graduate school—that the meaning of the basketball epiphany became apparent.

An English major at Princeton, I wanted to be a professor of literature. Reading and explicating the great works of human imagination—from Greek tragedies to Shakespeare—seemed like a good way to spend my working life. But my studies didn't illuminate what happened in the last five seconds of that game. Four years of the humanities and social sciences—reading widely in literature and philosophy, history and religion—didn't answer the two questions that the game in the Fieldston gym had left me with: What happened when the world as I knew it—planning and worrying, judging and fearing—momentarily dropped away? Could I access that state of being again and live differently?

In my senior year of college, I decided that if I was going to teach literature for the next several decades, I should first broaden my perspective. The year after college I volunteered in a program for troubled teens at Mt. Sinai Hospital in New York City and at a halfway house for schizophrenic young adults on Long Island. I loved this work and decided that I'd rather help people in pain than decode great books.

I went to graduate school to train to become a therapist rather than a literary critic, noticed that they sometimes overlap, discovered psychoanalysis, and was immediately hooked. Psychoanalysis demonstrated that there was a hidden depth and logic to even the most stubborn suffering and that through patient, disciplined, empathic awareness miraculous pathways could be constructed out of the prisons that held many of us captive.

At the same time, I began voraciously reading the classics of Eastern and Western psychology and spirituality. Buddha and Freud, Jung and Krishnamurti were my guides and mentors in my quest to illuminate what happened in the Fieldston gym. Existence became, for me, a question, and I immersed myself in plumbing its depths and fathoming its secrets.

But it wasn't until I participated in my first Buddhist meditation retreat in 1977 with renowned teachers Joseph Goldstein, Jack Kornfield, and Sharon Salzberg that I found myself on a path that illuminated that day on the basketball court and so much more.

The Gifts of the Dharma

The teachings of the Buddha gave me several priceless gifts, including a new way of looking within, which helped me see.

Worrying about a future that has never happened, replaying old hurts and wounds, cascading like a pinball from memories to fantasies to fears—the mind has a mind of its own. Even when we think we see clearly, we often observe life through a distorted lens. Our attention is scattered; we are "somewhere else," absent from our own lives and asleep to ourselves and to other people.

A mirror wiped clean: the experience of meditation. Meditation, the training of moment-to-moment attention, helped me begin to watch the workings of my own mind and become more aware of its wayward flights. By teaching me to hear what I listened to, see what I looked at, and taste what I ate, meditation showed me how asleep I was, how much life I had missed. Because of meditation I gained a heightened ability to be "here," to have a more whole-hearted presence and to be more receptive to the world—joining whatever I was doing in a deeper and richer way. I began to glimpse greater possibilities for awareness and clarity, freedom and compassion.

A psychiatrist once asked a teacher of Zen—Suzuki Roshi—what he thought of altered states of consciousness. "I'm just trying to help my students hear the birds sing" (Chadwick, 2001, p. 107), he replied. Paying attention helped me experience more life, and ordinary life took on a more sacred character.

The Buddha's teachings offered a way of celebrating daily life—and its wondrous gifts—including its beauty and marvels.

Buddhist ethical teachings—attention to speech and conduct, relationships and work—gave me a more systematic and less self-centered framework to live my ethics in everyday life: to speak, relate, and work in a way that caused less harm. Meditation also fostered a deeper level of compassion—an allegiance to the human family (and its non-human, furry compatriots)—rather than a narrow circle of family, friends, and colleagues.

As my meditation practice deepened my interests broadened, and I became more interested in bringing meditative practice to the world—in my case to the work I did as a psychoanalyst. Meditation practice and the Buddha's teachings gave me tools for living the insights I had on the basketball court—integrating them into how I worked as well as lived.

The Analyst's Couch and the Meditation Cushion

I sit in my office in New York City and stare at the statue of the Buddha on my windowsill. It is now over 45 years since I first participated in my first Buddhist meditation retreat and began practicing meditation. In the intervening years I became interested in integrating the wisdom of the Eastern meditative and Western psychotherapeutic traditions and illuminating the perils and possibilities of both paths. *Psychotherapy and Buddhism* (1996), *The Good Life* (2004), *The Art of Flourishing* (2009), and this book have been the partial fruit of that quest.

The five things meditative practice gave me—a heightened capacity for presence; a taste of an uncongealed and non-clinging mind; a deeper conception of compassion; an awareness of the possibility of wisdom; and a practice that nurtured improvisational living—have immeasurably transformed and enriched my life and my work.

As did psychoanalysis, which illuminated the mind in conflict, the characteristic challenges that human beings confront, and the ways we attempt to protect against and lessen emotional endangerment and pain. Psychoanalysis also aided me in being more interested in the truth of my patients' experiences rather than the correctness of my theories. And it provided a method—a special state of empathic, compassionate listening—and a special kind of self-reflective relationship to explore and midwife profound kinds of psychological transformation.

Psychoanalysis complemented my studies of meditation, yoga, and qigong, and revealed buried aspects of myself—including self-protective strategies that can be self-sabotaging—that the Asian wisdom traditions seemed to miss. From psychoanalysis, I learned about the seemingly inexhaustible human capacity for self-deception and the elaborate ways we all strive to lessen emotional pain.

The question animating my work over several decades has been: "How can I help people free themselves from the emotional prisons they construct to protect themselves?" My own interest in self-imprisonment and freedom began in high school. I grew up in an affluent, New York suburban community composed of men who were role models of what I didn't want to be, and women who seemed to sacrifice their authenticity in the quest for male affirmation, which further subjugated them and deepened their already substantial self-alienation.

The recognition of imprisonment and the experience of freedom formed the twin poles of the vision of psychology and spirituality that has informed my work as a therapist, teacher of psychology and meditation, and writer. Most people tend to highlight one and neglect the other—emphasizing that we have boundless possibilities (Positive Psychology, the Happiness movement, and pop psycho-spiritual gurus), or that we are enslaved (Western psychology and postmodern philosophy). I recognized, relatively early on in my career, that both are partially true and that we can't have one (call it "the light") without the other ("the shadow"). That would be like having a one-sided coin. Thus, either perspective presented alone is a half-truth. And a half-truth presented as the total truth is a lie, as my friend and teacher Joel Kramer used to say.

Bruce Lee, the legendary martial artist, provided unexpected guidance and inspiration in my ongoing quest to integrate the wisdom of "East" and "West" and create a psychology of health and wellness that didn't neglect psychoanalytic wisdom about the psychology of illness.

References

Chadwick, David. *Zen is Right Here: Teachings Stories and Anecdotes of Shunryu Suzuki*. Boston: Shambhala, 2001.

Rubin, Jeffrey B. *Psychotherapy and Buddhism: Toward an Integration*. New York: Plenum Press, 1996.

Rubin, Jeffrey B. *The Good Life: Psychoanalytic Reflections on Love, Ethics, Creativity, and Spirituality*. Albany: State University of New York Press, 2004.

Rubin, Jeffrey B. *The Art of Flourishing: A New East-West Approach to Staying Sane and Finding Love in an Insane World*. New York: Crown Archetype, 2009.

White, Patrick. *The Solid Mandala*. New York: Penguin Books. (Originally published 1966), 1983.

Yamada, Koun. *Zen: The Authentic Gate*. Translated by Maurice Shonen Walshe. San Francisco: Wisdom Publications, 2015.

2 Absorb What is Useful . . . Add What is Specifically Your Own

Bruce Lee and Me

Therapists, like the people they work with, sometimes contend with private demons. For many years I had a haunting nightmare: In the dead of night, I am being chased by a man who wants to kill me. I furiously pump my arms as I try to escape from him. No matter how hard I struggle to escape, he gets closer with each step. I feel terrified and helpless. And I think that I am soon going to die. I wake up with my jaw clenched and realize I was screaming.

For years I assumed that the dream represented my own intense self-criticism, which I inherited from my perfectionistic father—what Freud termed super-ego—and I thought the dream symbolized that I was chasing and attacking myself. A wonderful therapist emphasized a different aspect of the dream: "No one heard your screams," he said, but despite our collective efforts to understand it, the nightmare persisted—until I encountered Bruce Lee.

Bruce Lee. The name—and the visual image—conjure up waves of joy in the minds of a vast range of people from inner-city teenagers to middle-class adults. One of my friends said her 12-year-old son and her 79-year-old father both knew of—and loved—Bruce Lee.

An East Coast hoopster, who played basketball every waking moment in my youth when I wasn't reading or sleeping, I missed the heyday of Bruce Lee—the late 1960s to the early 1970s—and knew nothing about the "Little Dragon" and his martial arts exploits on the silver screen and in dojos on the West Coast. Yet later, his often-quoted advice "Utilize all ways and be bound by none," would become like a mantra to me.

A virtuoso martial artist, Lee attracted a group of American students after he immigrated to the United States from Hong Kong when he was a young adult in the early 1960s. The Chinese martial arts community in Oakland, California, demanded that he stop teaching students who weren't Chinese. Lee, who loved the martial arts and his heritage, refused because he wanted to teach any sincere person, regardless of race, gender, or ethnicity. He was issued an ultimatum: fight a challenger selected by his adversaries. If he was defeated, he must stop teaching. While he dispensed with his opponent in several minutes, he concluded that the fight took too long because he was

DOI: 10.4324/9781003604730-3

confined by the technique that he had mastered. He realized that traditional martial arts training and techniques were too rigid and unresponsive to the realities of the living moment and that he must be liberated from what he had become proficient at.

Lee, whose motto was "Research your own experience, absorb what's useful, reject what is useless and add what is specifically your own," studied as many martial and combat arts as he could, including traditional Chinese, Japanese, and Filipino systems, fencing, and the footwork of Muhammad Ali. He incorporated what was useful from each and discarded the rest.

In *The Tao of Jeet Kune Do*, Lee (1975) presented a devastating critique of the way martial arts were traditionally studied and practiced. He maintained that the vast majority of martial arts are specialists who strive to master one art, which they apply to every situation. This provides a framework and is reassuring. It also enslaves them. Substitute the word *therapists* for *martial artists* and Lee's point is just as applicable for psychotherapy.

In the mid-1980s, when I was in my 30s, I attended an all-day workshop in New York City on the philosophy and martial arts strategies of Bruce Lee. After the workshop I had a dream in which I was walking toward a bridge and saw a man kneeling down to tie his shoes. Out of the corner of my eye I noticed another man behind me, walking toward me. I knew that they were teaming up to rob me. I fought back and they ran away.

The nightmare of being chased never reoccurred.

Years later in my own therapy I realized that the dream was a flashback to trauma I had never processed and worked through: a concrete representation of an annihilating experience as an 8-year-old, when I was whipped with a belt by my father after he received a phone call that I had written something inappropriate on the back of a girl's class picture. Before that time, I was a playful, spontaneous kid, a fun-loving practical joker. After the whipping, my world of spontaneity and innocence ended and I became a "good" little buttoned-down boy, who was self-conscious and accommodating and strove to be an ideal self. Basketball was the only realm where I accessed an assertive, un-self-conscious me. The martial arts workshop helped me become reunited with the part of me that had been repressed after the trauma and allowed me to access normal aggression.

Intrigued and inspired by how Bruce Lee indirectly helped with the recurrent nightmare, I began studying his life and philosophy at the Princeton Academy of Martial Arts (PAMA) in 1995, under the tutelage of Sifu Rick Tucci and Sifu Jeff Jones, who taught Jun Fan gung fu, the foundation of Jeet Kune Do, the integrative and ever-evolving system fashioned by Bruce Lee and Guru Dan Inosanto, his close friend and main training partner. Sifu Rick and Sifu Jeff were students of Guru Dan, who had been given permission by him to teach. These studies provided a second, unexpected gift: a concrete method that inspired and supported my own quest to integrate the best of Eastern contemplative and somatic disciplines and Western psychotherapy, as well as anything else that deepened my craft and enhanced my capacity to help other people.

After I studied for a while with Sifu Rick and Sifu Jeff at PAMA, I participated in a weekend workshop with Guru Dan Inosanto. A renowned martial
artist and teacher with encyclopedic knowledge and experience, Guru Dan
had spent the intervening years after Bruce Lee's untimely death in 1973 continuing his friend's legacy by studying, learning, and fashioning an integrative
and ever-evolving approach to the martial arts and life. I spoke with Guru
Dan before the beginning of his workshop: "I am trying to do in psychotherapy what you and Si Jo Bruce Lee did in the martial arts. What were the
organizing principles you used to choose among the various arts that you
were exposed to, so that it wasn't a wild eclecticism?"

"Research your own experience and absorb what is useful, reject what is
useless, and add what is specifically your own," he replied, which I had read
in Bruce Lee's writings, but suddenly came alive in a more emotionally vivid
way. What he said next opened a new passageway: "It seems to me that therapy has three elements: a client, a therapist, and an environment. Since all
three are not always the same, therapy has to be different in each situation."

Bruce Lee and Dan Inosanto's integrative philosophy of being open to all
ways without clinging to any style, pattern, or mold—what the former called
"the way of no [set] way"—can be applied with stunning results to the training and practice of therapy. It provided me with a more systematic logic and
set of principles for what I had been attempting to do in therapy—integrating
the best of what I had studied (from psychoanalysis and meditation to qigong
and the martial arts) into a fluid and evolving framework that is customized
rather than standard-brand and attuned to the uniqueness of each situation
and the specific needs of each person.

I have a profound debt of gratitude to these pioneers for opening up new
pathways in integrative thinking and practice.

And I enjoy sleeping peacefully through the night.

Flow Rather Than Fight

During the Covid pandemic I reached out to my old teacher, Sifu Jeff Jones,
and began studying with him again. He had left Princeton Academy of Martial Arts and started his own school, Tri-State Kickboxing and Mixed Martial
Arts, in 2003. Since I trained with him in the mid-1990s my interests had
broadened from Buddhist meditation and Indian yoga to Chinese internal
martial arts and meditative and health practices such as *bagua* and qigong
(or Chi Kung, Chinese for "energy mastery"), a physical discipline involving deliberate movement and relaxed breathing, mental concentration and
visualization. Qigong is a corporal art and a form of Chinese internal exercise that can radically improve one's health and well-being. In addition, for
about nine years I had been studying a profound Russian holistic system of
self-exploration and health called *Systema*, and more recently begun training
in Brazilian jiu jitsu.

A superb teacher, who has become a good friend, Sifu Jeff resumed teaching
me Bruce Lee's Jun Fan gung fu and Kali, an integrative Filipino martial art that

Guru Dan Inosanto made popular. Sifu Jeff and I also shared a passion for what we call "JKD-ing it"—exploring how Bruce Lee's integrative philosophy of using all ways and being bound by none applies to various aspects of our lives from work and relationships to martial arts training and our own personal growth.

My studies with Sifu Jeff and my other teachers have been enormously fulfilling, as well as a continuing source of illumination and an invaluable and unexpected resource for practicing psychotherapy.

Teachers and students of martial arts and qigong know that devoted practice enhances concentration and focus, self-discipline and self-confidence. My immersion in both disciplines of transformation also led to greater somatic and emotional sensitivity and attunement—which fostered greater empathy, creativity, and intuition and expanded personal freedom and interpersonal adaptability. For me, the most surprising and inspiring discovery was that martial arts and qigong continually offered insights and metaphors that enriched my therapeutic work. With its attention to relaxed breathing even amid physical pain or fear and cultivation of exquisite bodily awareness and interpersonal attunement, Systema, for example, fostered a capacity to flow with—rather than fight, flee from, or freeze—challenging experiences and what normally overwhelms us. This has aided me in helping couples and individuals to be qualitatively more open to difficult feedback from their partners and to navigate trauma and other enslaving facets of their history rather than be emotionally allergic to it, panic at the first sign of demanding feelings, and attempt to vanquish them.

Systema for Life

"What would you do if your grandmother was attacked in Nazi Germany?" a member of the Valley Stream, Long Island Draft Board asked me in the fall of 1971. I was being interviewed about my application to be a conscientious objector. A pacifist, who took bugs outside as a kid rather than squish them, I was opposed to killing of any kind.

"No one—not you and not me—really knows what they will do when they are in danger," I said. "But you can hit someone over the head with a garbage can without killing them."

My pacifism was a sincere and heartfelt philosophical stance, arising out of reading Socrates and the Gospels, Thoreau and Gandhi, Martin Luther King and Daniel Berrigan in high school. I now realize it was also shaped by constructing a male identity on the shaky foundation of renouncing my father's rage.

My father had a vicious temper. I never knew when it would erupt. After one of his tirades when I was a teenager, I ran to my room, kneeled on the red and blue shag carpet on the floor, folded my hands in prayer and looked toward the ceiling of my room to the deity I was agnostic about: "Make me not an animal like my father and I'll believe in you," I said.

That was a fatal decision: I unconsciously linked healthy self-assertion, anger, and aggression with my father's temper. From then on, I tried to banish natural and necessary parts of being human and male. Anger, for example, can be invaluable feedback that you're being mistreated or emotionally hurt or disappointed, even threatened. If no one felt rage or discontent, there would have been no Civil Rights, feminist, or gay and lesbian rights movement. It took me several decades to realize the huge psychological cost of attempting to eliminate in myself what I associated with aspects of my father that terrified and disturbed me.

In a martial arts workshop in Toronto in 2016, I was partnered with an athletic and energetic instructor in his late 20s. I gently helped Tom to the ground as I performed a successful takedown. "You can help me up afterward, but you don't need to help me down," he said. It was a graphic physical illustration of the life-long emotional pattern of taking care of the other person and constraining my natural aggression.

My "solution" to my father's rage—mold myself into a choirboy who accommodated other people, fell asleep to himself, and suppressed aggression—was a band-aid. Like all makeshift "self-cures," it was brittle, unsustainable, and harmful. Fearing aggression and pushing it underground skewed and constrained my vision and freedom. What fed my tendency to deny myself—and what held in place my dysfunctional role in my biological family—were the twin pillars of pathological accommodation (Brandchaft, Doctors, & Sorter, 2010) and constrained self-assertion and aggression. And until I worked out the latter, I would forever be imprisoned within an unlocked cell that I was unable to leave.

Help came from an unexpected source—Systema, a holistic Russian system of self-exploration, healing, and combat drawn from centuries of monastic and martial traditions. Systema, which is Russian for "the system"—a way of being fostering self-knowledge—which is at once, a remarkable form of combat and self-preservation, and a profound spiritual path. For me, it shone a whole new light on the often-quoted line from Frederick Nietzsche's (1883–1891/1954) *Thus Spoke Zarathustra:* "There is more reason in your body than in your best wisdom."

Vladimir Vasiliev (2006), one of Systema's preeminent teachers and practitioners and author of several books including *Let Every Breath . . . Secrets of the Russian Breath Masters* describes it as a style that is "natural and free" and without a "rigid structure" or "strict rules." Responses are based on intuitive reactions. There are three components, according to Vladimir:

One: A body that is "free of tension, filled with endurance, flexibility, effortless movement and explosive potential."

Two: A "spirit or psychological state" that is "calm, free of anger, irritation, fear, self-pity, delusion, and pride."

Three: Movements that are "powerful and precise, instant and economical, spontaneous, subtle and diverse."

The foundational principle of Systema is "non-destruction." The goal, as Vladimir notes, "is to make sure that your training and your attitudes do no damage to the body or psyche of you or your partners." Systema is "designed to create, build and strengthen your body, your psyche, your family and your country," in Vladimir's view.

Pacifism is an admirable philosophy, but a fatally flawed one in a universe like ours. Gandhi could shame the moral conscience of the British. But boycotts and hunger strikes will not galvanize terrorists or fundamentalists or racists or American politicians who feel continually endangered to do the right thing. You can't shame someone who doesn't cherish life or have a conscience.

Defending ourselves from physical danger and emotional attacks becomes more imperative in a polarized world permeated by a politics of escalating hate. Hate never cures hate, as Christ and the Buddha knew—in fact, it only exacerbates it. But as an adult I have seen through my adolescent idealism and recognized that love often fails to lessen the meanness of the hard-hearted. And that puts many of us at a dangerous disadvantage and physically and emotionally vulnerable in a universe of seemingly endless animosity.

"We teach you to relax, not protect yourself," my Systema teacher, Edgars Cakuls, recently said in class. Experienced practitioners are calmer and more unperturbed, adaptable and resilient. And lethal. And that teaches you how to prevail in a variety of adverse situations—from facing an opponent with a knife, stick, or chain, to handling multiple attackers or coping with physical pain or fear. The goal of Systema, which is also a name for knowing yourself (*poznai sebia* in Russian), lie in a different direction.

It's lunchtime at a martial arts workshop in British Columbia in January 2017. I have traveled from New York to study with Igor Ponizov, a highly skilled and deceptively unassuming Systema instructor from Toronto. I am sitting next to him at lunch. He asks me how I am. I tell him about the deaths of my parents within ten days several months earlier. In the course of our conversation, he says: "The goal of Systema is to be a good person. Systema is a style of life." "Systema is life education, not [just] a martial art," Cakuls, another immensely talented and humble Systema instructor, recently said to me.

Systema is simple and straightforward—you move like an un-self-conscious child and respond in a natural and free manner—but it's not easy. Most martial arts emphasize techniques, which can be effective, but are often limiting, because they constrain responsiveness to the unique moment. Systema contains core principles—breathing, relaxing, adopting natural body positions, engaging in continuous movement, and blending with your partner (or opponent), based on sensitivity to them—rather than predetermined responses.

Studying Systema has been enormously challenging, as well as gratifying. Becoming a competent practitioner requires that we "unlearn" fundamental aspects of our emotional and physical conditioning—resisting and tightening under pressure; fighting or fleeing when attacked; thinking (instead of feeling) how to respond under duress. It is emotionally unsettling, as well as liberating, to defy instinctive habits that we take for granted. It challenges our pride—our sense of self-importance—which we fiercely cling to. The last thing Igor Ponizov said to me when I first trained with him in Toronto in 2015 was "Keep working on [lessening] pride in everyday life. Practice continuously and you will eventually see results."

Systema principles may initially sound (and feel) simplistic and elusive, but over time they prove to be profoundly real and eminently applicable to one's daily life. I saw this firsthand. My granddaughter is an avid and intrepid climber. A few years ago, a huge tree had fallen in my backyard. Juli, who was three, loved to walk across it. When she got to a rough patch with a steep drop on one side, she got nervous. "Breathe into your nose and out of your mouth," I said. I held her hand as she carefully traversed the tree. Whenever she subsequently faced a challenging physical or emotional situation, I would recommend the core Systema breathing technique. She took my suggestion seriously.

"Grandpa, the pavement is hot, and it hurts my feet," Juli, who was 6 at the time, said as we were walking toward an outdoor shower after a day at the beach.

"Me too, sweetie. We are almost there. What I do is exhale through the mouth hard when it hurts—*phew, phew, phew*. See if that helps."

"Grandpa, it works!" she replied a few seconds later.

That year, my then 7-year-old grandson, Gabe, got a nasty splinter. As Juli saw her older brother panic, she said: "Do the breathing, Gabe."

"The breathing," as well as numerous other Systema practices, have helped the three of us and countless students of Systema, handle everything from receiving a punch to the gut, to being thrown by another person, to facing an emotionally challenging situation.

Our highly conditioned self-protective reactions—fight, flee, or freeze—have an important survival purpose. They also hamper us under duress—causing us to tense and resist what scares or surprises us. Systema teaches a fourth way: *flow*. Systema trains one to respond to whatever life brings by breathing, relaxing, and creatively responding.

Imagine that someone grabs your right arm. Because of pride or tension, fear or injury, you tighten and resist and pull it away. Your reaction creates what Systema calls a "bridge" to the other person, which heightens his tension and causes him to tug harder. Your tension and resistance and pain mounts, and so does his. It's a mutually escalating negative cycle that is a microcosm of what happens between hostile spouses, citizens, and even nations.

In Systema you never fight a problem at its origin. For example, if your partner grabs your wrist and twists your arm, you comply, breathe, relax your arm and wrist, and realign whatever parts of your body are bent such as your shoulder and hips.

Now imagine the same scenario except you drop your hips and relax your shoulder and let the other person pull you. "Thank you for the gift; relax and don't care; feel it and don't think what to do," is the counterintuitive attitude my teacher recommends. Your opponent will feel no tension and resistance from you, and you will feel no pain. And they will be emotionally confused and physically thrown off-balance by your emotional and physical relaxation, which was unexpected. And this provides what my teacher calls a "pathway" to extricate oneself from the problem and the danger.

As I became more familiar and comfortable with relaxing under pressure and regaining physical balance with a partner in class, Systema principles organically came into my work as a psychotherapist. "Don't make a bridge to your wife when she is hostile," I say to an easy-going man who is continually verbally attacked by his spouse. "Restore yourself using breathing, and then reengage with her from that place, which will be more constructive."

A few weeks later he told me: "Initially my wife was thrown off-balance when I didn't 'add logs to the fire.' She had nothing to fight against. No punching bag to hit. Then she softened and was more reasonable." His relaxed and non-contentious response to her helped her become aware of her tone and anger.

We live in a world that has a talent for arousing fears. We are afraid of many things: falling behind and losing our jobs or homes; not measuring up and not being loved; nuclear war or race riots; and being persecuted or ostracized because of ethnicity, religion, or gender.

"Train fear every day," Igor said when I studied with him. "Every day."

"Fear is For Others" was emblazoned on Michael's tee shirt above a silk screen of Bruce Lee. He sought psychotherapy after he was brutalized in a sneak attack in a bar, which he blamed himself for, and felt humiliated by.

"There *is* fear," I said when I saw his shirt, which was my shorthand for "There *is* fear within you." The wider resonance of my remark—that we are all afraid (and experience anger, guilt, and shame and every other emotion)— only struck me later.

"It was a sign of great weakness," he informed me. "That would never have happened to a really skilled Systema practitioner," he opined. (He had asked me about self-defense and martial arts when we first met and was familiar with Systema).

It seemed to me that what fueled his shame was a fantasy that he should be beyond fear.

"A really skilled Systema practitioner might anticipate—or even preempt—a surprise attack," I said. "And they are trained to relax in the face of it, which greatly decreases the tension and pain. But my teacher is also constantly reminding me that it is not a question of getting beyond fear, which is unavoidable, but gradually training oneself to recover from it more quickly."

Systema has enriched my life, as well as my work. It showed me a pathway beyond the stultifying options of mindlessly rejecting qualities associated with my father or imitating his terrifying rage. There was a middle-way between violence and self-effacement. I could be strong without being destructive; tough yet kind; assertive without being angry.

Learning to defend oneself, yet inflict the minimum of harm, is an indispensable tool in a world of escalating cruelty and malevolence. I am also grateful to Systema because it has been a doorway into self-healing and self-transformation.

The process of growing up and aging warps us. We develop in one-sided ways physically and emotionally. We tend to cultivate our strengths and ignore and neglect our weaknesses. And this perpetuates and exacerbates our imbalances. Our bodies as well as our minds reveal the impact—overuse injuries, chronic stiffness, and physical constriction.

I begin my day with Systema breathing and relaxation exercises and self-restorative practices. I breathe through the whole body; direct breath into areas of tension and injuries; extend the breath; breathe with the minimum of exertion; tighten and relax each area of the body, stretch tendons; practice voluntary control over individual segments of the body; do drills to cultivate fine motor coordination of the hands and shoulders; synchronize breath with movements; do self-massage and exercises to trigger and relax in the face of fear and so forth.

Systema is an exquisite training in awareness and sensitivity. It cultivates enhanced attunement to internal physical processes and emotions. This has helped me heal stubborn leg injuries, expand physical capacities, create more harmony between my mind and body, access relaxation amid stressful situations; and heighten awareness in everyday life—especially attunement to hidden emotional and bodily tensions—for example, the constriction of my breathing or the tightening of my shoulders when subliminal worry or fear arises. Apprehension tends to sneak up on us and affect our body and our mind before we are even aware of its existence. After practicing Systema I more readily notice the first instance of feelings—when they arise as somatic sensations—which helps me understand and work more skillfully with challenging ones, personally and as a psychotherapist.

Systema has been a mirror reflecting back deeper psychological conditioning. Basketball was my first love. Not only has it been a life-long passion; it saved my life. It was a sanctuary from the madness in my family that threatened to annihilate me.

Basketball was also my first meditation teacher, as I said in Chapter 1. It taught me how to focus and it gave me many of my deepest spiritual insights.

Basketball was imprisoning as well as liberating: it entrapped me within the ultimately self-undermining project of trying to be the best and justify my existence. The quest for perfection honed excellence and fostered positive self-regard. But that was an impossible dream and a misguided one, for as long as the focus was excelling, instead of simply playing, a sense of failure was continuous. For all of its virtues, basketball perpetuated and left untouched emotional conditioning that I needed to transform.

The chief obstacles to doing Systema are pride (= self-importance) and fear, tension and thinking. They all interfere with sensitivity. The principles underlying Systema—breathe, relax, regain your natural physical structure, keep moving, and blend with your partner or opponent—can be difficult to execute. Not because they are complex, but because they challenge powerful unconscious psychological conditioning, as I suggested earlier.

At first, I assumed that my frustration with myself in learning and practicing Systema was endemic to becoming proficient in such a complex discipline. But I later realized that it was caused by my judging my imperfections and mistakes instead of simply learning from them. Unsurprisingly, the same conditioning that haunted me when I played basketball emerged during Systema training—the pressure to excel; the drive to be the best, the frustration when I had trouble learning something—which hindered my mastery and progress. But unexpectedly, and for the first time, I saw this pattern with crystalline clarity. And that has been a doorway into transforming the judging mind.

"In class and at workshops, think like a teacher," Igor said as we parted in British Columbia. "How would you teach differently?" I had been doing that without recognizing it, but until he said that I didn't realize the larger changes that Systema was generating.

Some years ago, I wanted to integrate yoga into my work. I drew on yogic breathing in my practice of psychotherapy, but I wanted to try to incorporate more aspects of yoga. Carl Horowitz, a yoga teacher and friend, recommended I read Gary Kraftsow's *Yoga for Transformation* (2002), and each day practice a different protocol he had for working with emotional problems. In addition, he suggested that a few days a week I spontaneously improvise with my own practice—taking what I had learned over several decades and experimenting based on what I needed in the moment. It was a great suggestion. But I had trouble doing it: I couldn't let go of the routines I had learned and just experiment and play.

Each week I attend two Systema classes and do two intensive private sessions with my teacher. Five other days I practice Systema on my own, and experiment and improvise each time. Systema training helped me access an improvisatory spirit I use in my psychotherapy practice, but that was inhibited with yoga.

"How is Systema?" my Zen teacher, Lou Mitsunen Nordstrom, used to ask me every Wednesday when we spoke. Each week I shared discoveries and insights.

"Systema takes Zen where it doesn't—and would like to—go," he said. "Zen students often have great difficulty taking Zen off of the cushion and into their lives. Systema is embodied Zen."

I experienced this firsthand.

Self-consciousness is a universal illness, according to Zen. Our reflective consciousness—our ability to step back and analyze our experience—is a wonderful capacity. It also creates a separation and a gap between our mind and body and self and other. Instead of greeting life directly, wholeheartedly, and freshly, like children, we approach it from a distance, indirectly. We lead second-hand lives. We listen to music but don't hear it; we eat food without tasting—let alone savoring—it. That is enormously self-alienating.

An experience I had training with Jamie Lippiatt, a Systema instructor in Toronto provided a glimpse of an alternative. "What would you like to work on?" Jamie, a 30-something black belt in Krav Maga and a 2007 Canadian jiu jitsu champion, asked me in the summer of 2015. "Healthy aggression," I say. I tell him about my father's temper and my own inhibited aggression. After doing some preliminary breathing, movement, and relaxation exercises he grabs me in a bear hug. "Try to escape," he says. We are about the same weight and height. I can't budge him. "Try again," he says. Same results. "Walk across the room," he says. I do. A strange thing happens: I easily drag him. "Did you change the pressure?" I ask. "Nope," he says. We do the same drill again. Same results. He gets me in another bear hug. "Try to escape," he says. I can't. "Pick up something from the ground," he says. As I bend down, I feel him leaning over my right shoulder. I turn slightly and he falls to the mat. "Reach for your keys on the ground," he says. I don't have any keys on the ground, but I know what he means. I bend as if I was going to pick up an item from the ground and he is again leaning precariously over my right shoulder. I turn slightly and he falls to the ground. I "escape" because I am un-self-conscious.

There's a concept in Zen and the martial arts called "no-mind" (*mushin* in Japanese)—awareness-without-self-consciousness. It's a state of mind and being in which one is alert and receptive, with attention not resting in any place in particular. Enormous freedom and creativity can emerge from such an unfettered mind.

"Systema teaches how to 'drop the mind,'" I tell my Zen teacher, "which accesses the body's natural intelligence." An empath who was trained to dismiss his own feelings and accommodate other people, Systema helped me regain my birthright of valuing my experience. "Systema ushered in a more experiential way of living," I added. "Because of Systema, I am in my body more in daily life. No-minded living has resulted in greater moment-to-moment awareness of my feelings. And this has been invaluable in navigating my family, contemporary life, and psychotherapy."

"Systema is a body mysticism," my Zen teacher replied. "But you have had an enigmatic relationship with your body."

"Conflictual, not enigmatic," I say. "Sports have been my inroad into meditation and mindful living. But the trauma of my family pulled me into my head. I was both attuned to and separated from, my body. I lived more in my head. Systema has brought me back to my body."

"What I have wanted for you is to get out of your head and into your body."

The home I yearned for was closer than I ever realized. Getting into my body provided it.

References

Brandchaft, Bernard, Shelley Doctors, & Dorienne Sorter. *Toward an Emancipatory Psychoanalysis: Brandchaft's Intersubjective Vision*. New York: Routledge, 2010.

Kraftsow, Gary. *Yoga for Transformation: Ancient Teachings and Practices for Healing the Body, Mind, and Heart*. New York: Penguin Compass, 2002.

Lee, Bruce. *The Tao of Jeet Kune Do*. Valencia, CA: Black Belt Books, 1975.

Nietzsche, Friedrich. *Thus Spoke Zarathustra*. Translated by Walter Kaufmann. New York: Random House, 1954. (Originally published 1883–1891).

Vasiliev, Vladimir. *Let Every Breath . . . Secrets of the Russian Breath Masters*. Toronto: Russian Martial Art, 2006.

3   One Size Never Fits All

The Birthday Party Nobody Attended

A patient of mine, Jaden, a therapist-in-training, was in a class on psychotherapy. Her teacher, a therapist, told the following story. A male client, a tremendously isolated single adult, with a life-long pattern of depriving himself, came into a therapy session on his birthday with two ice-cream cones, one for the therapist. Not only was his therapist the only person he really talked to, but therapy had helped him begin to value and take care of himself. For him this has been revolutionary, and he was deeply grateful.

The therapist assumed that the client's gift was an indirect, symbolic expression of sexualized feelings—and that by accepting the cone she would be breaking the sacred therapeutic rules and acting out a destructive scenario instead of exploring and illuminating it—so she avoided what she thought was a seduction and didn't accept the patient's gift.

The cone began melting in the patient's hands, creating a mess. The therapist tried to explore why the patient *wanted* to create a mess in her office. The patient was stunned.

He was also humiliated and deflated by "the birthday party that nobody attended."

"Why didn't she just take the cone and explore what it meant?" Jaden asked me.

"That's an interesting question," I said. "What do you think?"

"She didn't want to interfere with the patient bringing into therapy his habitual ways of thinking about himself and relating to other people arising from significant interactions with parents, siblings, and authority figures from the past—what Freud called the transference," Jaden said. "If she took the cone, it would contaminate the environment, and she couldn't explore the meaning of the transference to the patient."

"Why not?" I asked.

"If you had a physical illness and your doctor took blood from you to test, you would not want that sample tainted by the doctor's (or a lab technician's) blood," she said. "In order to determine what was in your blood, the sample must be just your own blood."

DOI: 10.4324/9781003604730-4

"In the case of complex emotional states," Jaden continued, "the patient must be allowed to speak of what is troubling them—to 'give blood' without contamination from an outside source, such as the therapist's judgment, opinions, and personal life. So, although the therapist may seem to be aloof or distant, or an unreadable cipher, what the therapist is really doing is being a blank page the patient can 'write' their own experiences on. This shows the therapist the truest picture of what is going on with the patient. The therapist knows that what is coming from the patient, for example, the expectation that the therapist will be judgmental, is transferred onto the therapist from the patient's own earlier life. If that therapist took the cone, it might have 'contaminated' the clean atmosphere of the therapeutic environment," she concluded.

"You know what the therapist—and you—are assuming?" I asked.

Jaden is silent but is staring intensely.

"Something very *un*-psychoanalytic—that if the therapist is not neutral, she'll interfere with the emergence of the patient's transference. But you don't so easily stop or dilute transference," I replied. "If transference is the way formative events from the past cause us to miss the freshness of the present, then the patient, like the rest of us, is going to express his transference anyway. It's inevitable."

"What would you have done?" Jaden asked.

"The patient was a highly isolated man who was deeply grateful to his therapist for helping him come out of his self-protective shell. I would have graciously accepted his gift and heartily thanked him for his gratitude. Then I would have wished him a very happy birthday. Then I would have enjoyed the gift with him *and* explored its potential meanings."

"Potential *meanings*?" my client asked.

"One way of thinking about therapy," I said, "is that the therapist has a dictionary of what things mean—trees are penises, boxes are vaginas—which they consult when the patient speaks or acts. Everything has a predetermined significance that the therapist knows in advance. From this perspective the therapist is a 'customs official' who knows ahead of time what is 'foreign' or 'illegal' and is vigilant that nothing dangerous is smuggled in. Freud demonstrated that this approach is completely false and inadequate."

"It's as if therapy is a war or battle and the therapist holds the fort against the invasion," my client said.

"Exactly," I replied. "In reality, the cone could mean many things ranging from sexual imagery to the expression of gratitude."

I continued, "In his book *Psychoanalytic Theory, Therapy, and the Self*, Harry Guntrip (1971) put it like this: 'Theory is a useful servant but a bad master.' When you assume you know ahead of time what something means—or whether it's detrimental (or helpful) to the therapy (or the person's life)—you run the risk of treating the wrong person; the patient you've created in your mind; instead of the person in front of you. The problem with this approach is that the therapist's preconceptions—actually biases—may not coincide with the understanding of the person they are working with. Not only does the therapist miss the patient, but they become locked into—and enslaved by—whatever she already believes."

"What happened by not accepting the gift?" Jaden asked.

"The therapist was not neutral—which it is impossible to be—and humiliated the patient. And the patient may have felt hopeless about being understood and going deeper with this therapist, as well as shamed and silenced."

"Here is another way of thinking about therapy," I said. "The therapist often doesn't know what something means. Clients teach us what things mean *to them* based on their experience and reactions. The therapist is then more like a "jazz improviser" who is grounded in the fundamentals of human development and the therapeutic process and needs to creatively spring from that based on the demands of the present moment. From that perspective the therapist could accept the gift *and* investigate its unique implications."

Our Most Important Task

If one size never fits all, we need to individualize the treatment and meet people where they are. How do we do this, and what gets in the way?

From Buddhism to behaviorism, Western culture is permeated with the implicit as well as explicit, search to transcend the dizzying intricacy of inner life and external existence. In the face of the nearly limitless complexity of both there is a powerful human tendency to reduce and narrow down, which is emotionally and intellectually reassuring because it creates an apparent order—an internal and external world that, as I discussed in *The Good Life* (2004), can be mapped.

There is a tension in psychoanalysis between its liberatory and constricting tendencies. At its best moments, psychoanalysis is *the art of the idiographic*, interested in the unique individual. On the other hand, psychoanalysts all too often fall into formulaic and generalized thinking and theorizing, which eclipses the individual. Freud's theory of dream practice illustrates this tension.

In his magnum opus, *The Interpretation of Dreams*, Freud (1900) wrote that previous investigators of dreams adopted one of two typical approaches: they assumed that there was a singular symbolic meaning to a dream, or they used a standardized formula for decoding the meaning. In the "decoding method," dreams are viewed as "a kind of cryptography in which each sign can be translated into another sign having a known meaning, in accordance with a fixed key." Freud critiques this approach because "the same piece of content may conceal a different meaning when it occurs in various people or various contexts" and "every element in a dream can, for purposes of interpretation, stand for its opposite just as easily as for itself." The meaning of a dream, according to Freud, is discerned not by translating the dream into the *a priori* meaning and "fixed-key" of a "dream-book," but by eliciting the dreamer's unique associations. Freud's method "imposes the task of interpreting upon the dreamer him [or her] self. It is not concerned with what occurs to the interpreter in connection with a particular element of the dream, but with what occurs to the dreamer."

An important exception to this occurs when the analyst determines that the dream contains what Freud terms *symbols*, by which he means elements of the dream that indirectly represent latent dream thoughts, which are not derived from the day residue, are not revealed by free associations, and must be decoded by the analyst.

> As contrasted with other dream-elements, a fixed meaning may be attributed to them [symbols]. . . since we know how to translate these symbols and the dreamer does not . . . it may happen that the sense of a dream may at once become clear to us as we have read the text of the dream, even before we have made any effort at interpreting it, while it still remains an enigma to the dreamer himself.
>
> (1933, pp. 12–13)

"The concept of a symbol," Freud admits in *The Interpretation of Dreams*, (1900)

> cannot at present be sharply delimited; it shades off into such notions as those of replacement or representation, and even approaches that of an illusion . . . You see, then, that a symbolic relation is a comparison of a quite special kind, of which we do not as yet clearly grasp the basis, though perhaps we may later arrive at some indication of it.

Freud continues by recommending a "combined technique" when dealing with "those elements of the dream-content which must be recognized as symbolic." The "combined technique," on the one hand, "rests on the dreamer's associations" and on the other hand, "it fills the gap from the interpreter's knowledge of symbols."

Melvin B. Lansky wrote in "The Legacy of *The Interpretation of Dreams*" (1992) that Freud does not specify *how* the analyst knows that a particular facet of the dream is a symbol, rather than something that needs to be examined afresh using the associative method. He also does not provide any criteria to validate such a decision. That this can open the door to interpretive confusion is suggested by Freud's recognition that "the presence of symbols in dreams not only facilitates their interpretation but also makes it more difficult." One crucial difficulty is hermeneutical reductionism, by which I mean that the analyst, to use Freud's image in a different but compatible context, "interprets *into*" the analysand's utterances what cannot be interpreted *from* them and thus assimilates the uniqueness of the dream material into the "fixed meaning" of their generalized theories.

The Freudian theory of dream practice—with its clashing conceptions of the associational and symbolic approach to the ideographic dream material— both illustrates and provides resources for transforming the tension between the constricting and liberating dimensions of psychoanalysis. The presumption that the analyst can ascertain that particular material in a dream is symbolic, and therefore can be interpreted without the dreamer's associations funnels the radically novel content of the dream into the preexisting categories of the analyst's dream meanings—the "fixed-key" of their personal "dream-book"— and thus interferes with the emergence of the analysand's unique subjectivity. Being a midwife to the psychological birth of the inimitable person we are working with is the most important task we have.

References

Freud, Sigmund. *The Interpretation of Dreams*. Standard Edition, 4–5: xxxiii–627. London: Hogarth Press, 1900.

Freud, Sigmund. *Revision of the Theory of Dreams*. Standard Edition, 22: 5–30. London: Hogarth Press, 1933.

Guntrip, Harry. *Psychoanalytic Theory, Therapy, and the Self*. New York: Basic Books, 1971.

Lansky, Melvin B. "The Legacy of *The Interpretation of Dreams*." In *Essential Papers on Dreams*, edited by Melvin Lansky, 3–31. New York: New York University Press, 1992.

Rubin, Jeffrey B. *The Good Life: Psychoanalytic Reflections on Love, Ethics, Creativity, and Spirituality*. Albany: State University of New York Press, 2004.

4 The Psychotherapist as Jazz Improviser
A Walk on the Wild Side

"Can we take a walk?"

Roger's question was not as easy to answer as one might imagine.

Short and slight, Roger was an extremely intelligent and poetic man in his early 30s, who had been referred to me by a psychiatrist after he believed rays were being beamed into the bus he was on. He had been diagnosed several years before with schizophrenia (literally "split or cut mind"), after he claimed that there was a governmental plot afoot and ran screaming through the streets in the middle of the night in the Midwestern town where he attended graduate school. He was hospitalized, placed on anti-psychotic medication, and he returned home a defeated man, to live out his days with his elderly socialist parents.

Schizophrenia is a name that is as dreaded in the mental health sphere as cancer is in the world of medicine. It often conjures up images of people talking to themselves on the locked wards of state psychiatric hospitals, on public transportation, and on city streets, and of doing irrational and destructive things.

Before responding to Roger my mind flashed for a moment on the three books on my desk I had just finished reading. One was about a Tibetan Buddhist teacher who had slept with his students even though he knew that he had AIDS. The second one, *Turning the Wheel: American Women Creating the New Buddhism* (Boucher, 1988), was a collection of personal accounts of women who had been harmed by spiritual teachers: in 1983 five out of six of the most famous and esteemed Zen masters in the United States—supposedly enlightened beings who had achieved self-realization and were exemplars of the highest human development—had sexually exploited female students, stolen funds from the spiritual communities they led, and, in the case of at least two, abused alcohol. The third was a book that attempted to integrate Eastern spiritual and Western psychological perspectives on the human condition. The author had attempted to map everything from schizophrenia to mysticism on a single, linear grid. Human development, he proposed, was like a spectrum of light, with various aspects ranging from psychosis to mystical

DOI: 10.4324/9781003604730-5

awareness. Schizophrenics need drugs, not therapy, the author confidently concluded, and mystics were beyond both therapy and the rest of us, exemplifying the highest states of awareness and morality.

"What would you hope to gain by walking?" I asked in response to Roger's question.

"An opportunity to test my paranoia," he replied. "I could tell you how I am perceiving people in the world, and you could give me feedback."

"Do you see any downside to trying this?" I asked, thinking for a moment about my psychoanalytic training, which would have answered his request with a question ("Why do you want to walk?") and insisted that we never leave the office.

"No," he said.

"Well then let's try it," I said, getting up from my chair, not sure about the wisdom of our joint decision but influenced by Thelonius Monk's truism: "Jazz is freedom."

We walked out of my office. About 50 feet from the door, a group of teenage girls congregated near a corner. I could hear their laughter. "They are making fun of me," Roger said.

"How do you know?" I asked.

He was silent.

"I get the impression that they are not very aware of our existence," I said. "And if they are laughing at us, it is probably at my outfit." He glanced at me, saw that everything was intact, and laughed at my attempt at self-deprecation.

"Do you want to get a bite to eat?" Roger asked. He was usually very shy and self-effacing and never asked anything from anyone—so I viewed his request as a rare and deeply constructive attempt to both connect with me and express what he needed. But I feared that our experiment had crossed the line and gone too far—a walk on the therapeutic wild side.

We entered a modest Middle Eastern restaurant with pictures of Israel on the menus and several large video games against one of the walls. It was the mid-1980s. Without cell phones it was pretty quiet. We ordered food and then talked—about his life, and his hopes and fears.

When we were finished eating, I stood up and walked to the garbage so that I could throw away my plastic fork and knife. Roger interrupted me and asked why I was throwing away my utensils. "Because I am finished eating," I said, not sure what he was getting at.

"Do you know that that is ecologically unsound?" he asked. He was more surprised than judgmental.

To think about plastic forks and knives may be to miss what was most important about Roger's comment. He worried about not polluting the environment, not because he was "paranoid," and thought it would contaminate the world, but because he believed that each of us were "planet stewards" whose responsibility was to "preserve and protect the welfare of each other and the earth."

I thought of the spiritual biographies I had been reading as well as the two other books on my desk. The spiritual teachers in them were idealized for their wisdom and compassion. But Roger's sense of responsibility for the world raised a question for me about whether there is a troubling tension when gurus preach humanistic ideals while at the same time treating their ideal-hungry disciples like commodities.

I had no doubt that Roger was in agony. There had been a tendency, since the 1960s—especially among the anti-psychiatry movement—to glorify schizophrenics. Some writers viewed schizophrenia as a romantic refuge from the insanity of everyday life and claimed schizophrenics were the harbingers of freedom; liberated from the cultural shackles that bind us all. But Roger knew on a minute-to-minute basis a darker dark than either I, or the champions of the "wisdom" of psychosis, have ever encountered. Inside he faced a terrifying civil war—what he called "The Illness"—that I wouldn't want to celebrate.

Yet, despite his inner demons he walked gently upon the earth. He was kind and decent. As far as I could tell, and I knew a lot about him, he did not exploit anyone, what the yogic tradition calls *ahimsa*, variously translated from Sanskrit as non-harming and consideration for all living beings. And he tried with a ferocity, which I deeply respected, not to pass his pain onto anyone else. I wished that he would not feel so trapped and terrorized and that he could experience the closeness and intimacy to other human beings that he both desperately needed and perceived as so dangerous. But I had no doubt that he was more moral than many of the esteemed spiritual masters I had been reading about.

Excess often leads to disaster, as the promiscuous gurus demonstrate. One of the greatest lessons of my psychoanalytic training was the virtue of conducting therapy by an established set of rules that created and maintained for my patients a safe and protected therapeutic environment. Because of my training I was cautious and conservative. I became like a skilled customs official who knows ahead of time what is illegal and what shouldn't be smuggled in. There is great value to this stance. Boundaries give structure and stability and safety. They also protect the autonomy of patients.

But the "road of excess," as William Blake wrote in "The Marriage of Heaven and Hell" (1793/1970) can also lead "to the palace of wisdom." A walk on the wild side can court disaster—like when unscrupulous gurus or therapists sexually exploit people they are supposed to help and guide—because it often leads to impulsive and self-destructive behavior that harms other people, as well as us. But when we always play it safe, we may miss a lot of life.

I wouldn't walk or eat with most patients and it's not something I'd recommend to younger colleagues. But my sojourn with Roger led me deeper into his inner world and showed me the terror and humanity that he didn't fully bring into the safe and controlled haven of my office. I doubt I would have learned certain vital things about his soul, if I had not walked into his world and seen it through his eyes.

I thought back to Guru Dan's seemingly throwaway comment that "therapy has three elements—a client, a therapist, and an environment—and since all three are always different, therapy has to be different in every situation."

It is generally assumed that therapy always occurs in the same environment—the therapist's office. This is usually the case. With Roger the variable that changed was where we met—we walked outside—and it made all the difference.

References

Blake, William. "The Marriage of Heaven and Hell." In *Selected Poems*, edited by Peter Butter, 46–58. London: Dent, 1970. (Originally published 1793).

Boucher, Sandy. *Turning the Wheel: American Women Creating the New Buddhism*. San Francisco: Harper & Row, 1988.

5 The Incomparable Power of Human Understanding
Searching for Emotional Sanity Underneath the Madness

"I feel dead, like a mannequin," Roger said as our session began many years ago. He spoke by turns, haltingly and frenetically. Toward the end of the conversation, Roger suddenly shared a fantasy of getting up from his chair, running into the street, and crashing against a slow-moving car.

A variety of questions might arise as you contemplated the scenario Roger envisioned. Was he: Depressed? Suicidal? Hallucinating? Angry? High on drugs? I remember asking myself what he was trying to accomplish, which made me wonder if he was attempting to save and heal rather than destroy himself. I wondered, as Roger spoke during our session, if feeling lifeless and inert was safer for him than being constantly terrorized by delusions and hallucinations. Emily Dickinson was not alone in reminding us of the wisdom in apparent madness.

"Would slamming into the car create sensation, and would sensation make you feel real and alive?" I asked.

"Yes," he replied, suddenly more animated.

"Is feeling alive (with the risk of physical endangerment), preferable to feeling 'dead like a mannequin?'" I continued.

Roger brightened up, no longer looking lifeless and inert, and proceeded to enlighten me as to why and how he felt "psychologically dead."

Roger was one of the most courageous people I have ever met. He once told me that he was so vulnerable to things outside of him—sights, sounds, and people—that he was like a "cell without a membrane," raw, open, profoundly unprotected in a dangerous world. He faced a never-ending battle not to go crazy. At the end of our first session, several years earlier, he leaned forward and nearly whispering, asked if I would treat him using only intensive psychotherapy without forcing him to take drugs and become a "zombie."

"Let's try it and be honest about how it goes," I said, not sure if I was giving him a shot at a life or signing his death sentence.

The hell that Dante never envisioned in *The Divine Comedy*, the journey through the cave of madness—confronting and ultimately surmounting the various conspiracies that haunted Roger—had created a deep bond between us. From the day we did walking meditation on a local boardwalk overlooking

DOI: 10.4324/9781003604730-6

the ocean, not stopping until the inner terrorists no longer hijacked his mind, to the day we braved the Kafkaesque world of motor vehicles and he got his driver's license—we had moments of exhilaration and terror as we struggled to free him from the annihilating forces that threatened to deprive him of the chance of having a life of his own.

For Roger there were grave dangers associated with feeling alive. During a session, several months into treatment he began to get angry with me, but immediately squelched it. I asked him why he cut off his emotions.

"My feelings are like 'nuclear waste,' and they could 'contaminate' a weak and vulnerable world," he said.

I learned that when Roger was 18 years old, he tried, for the first time in his life, to separate from his dad, an overbearing intellectual man who was devoted to socialist politics and high culture and carve out his own life. As a result, Roger was increasingly at odds with his father, whose approval—which was never forthcoming—still meant the world to him. While Roger longed for the appreciation of his remote father, he felt compelled to test the unwritten limits of his family and have his own voice. "I hate you! I hope you die," Roger said to his father one day in anger.

His father was crushed and began crying and shaking after Roger's expression of anger. Roger felt horrible that he had hurt his father. That moment may have been more debilitating for Roger than it was for Dad. It strangled his spirit and hindered his natural expression of emotions.

For teenagers to be able to manage their genuine feelings—including, but not limited to hate—which are a natural part of healthy emotional development, the people in their lives need to be able to contain and survive them. Otherwise, these feelings will seem too dangerous—like nuclear waste.

When our parents can't handle our outbursts, we develop distorted ideas about our own dangerousness. We think we are despicable or burdensome or poisonous.

After his father's crushing reaction to his expression of hostility, Roger developed the deadly idea that he was "toxic," and other people were excessively fragile. His natural aggression and assertion were repressed and they festered. He began to see the world as if it was like his father—incapable of handling his genuine feelings. So, he put himself in "lockdown"—moving through the world in a highly controlled, excessively timid, and self-effacing way—imprisoned within his fear of damaging other people through his words and actions. He walked through the world as if he didn't want to take up any space.

And this might have been why he "put a bomb" in my filing cabinet. Several years into our therapy, Roger was terrified at the beginning of our session. I noticed him looking at my filing cabinet. I had no idea why.

"There's a bomb in the filing cabinet," he blurted out.

"Tell me more," I said.

He was silent for a while. I remained silent.

"I'm very angry at you," he burst out. "I guess I want to blow you up."
I was silent.
He was silent.
"We didn't meet last week," he said at last.
Speaking more slowly—and looking palpably relieved—he said: "There's no bomb in there anymore."
The use of the word "bomb" was no accident; it represented his emotional reaction to my disappointing him. He was terrified his feelings would "decimate" us and destroy our relationship.
From what we could reconstruct, Roger's problems actually began much earlier than when his father couldn't handle his aggression. In elementary school, Roger remembered believing that aliens were trying to steal parts of the encyclopedia he was trying to read. As I got to know Roger, I learned that his mother, a self-involved and oblivious artist, alternately neglected and intruded on her only child. She either left Roger too much to his own devices—forcing him to handle the torment he went through with bullies in elementary school and high school on his own—or barged in on him and tried to run his life. She was more interested in painting and reading literature than mothering her son.
For example, when he complained to her about the roof leaking in the living room, she ignored him and told him she was going to be studying James Joyce's *Finnegan's Wake*. The roof never got repaired until Roger hired a roofer to fix it. When Roger's mother did focus on her son it was in an excessively intrusive and cold manner. When he tried to talk with her about his feelings, she invalidated them—telling him what he should feel and "gas-lighting" him; undermining his belief in the reality of his own perceptions. Roger identified with Gregor Samsa, Kafka's infamous salesman in "The Metamorphosis," who woke up one morning to find himself transformed into an insect, who was incredibly vulnerable to being trampled on.
To provide an accurate picture of my ten-year journey with Roger through the caverns of madness I would have to be a Dostoevsky and Proust rolled into one. But if I had to try to give you a flavor of what happened I would stress several things.
Belief in the validity of one's sense of reality is essential to the development of a sense of self. The empathic attunement of one's caregivers is crucial to the gradual development of a child's trust in their perceptions and feelings. When this is absent or undependable, the child's belief in her own personal reality is undermined and vulnerable to disintegration. Difficult situations later in life may lead such a person to fragmentation. In a desperate attempt at self-healing, the person may develop delusional ideas that symbolically express what is endangering them.
As I witnessed, validated, and illuminated Roger's experiences and perceptions of reality—including various delusions—a deep bond developed between us. This was a rollercoaster ride. There were many times when our

work stalled or derailed, either because I misunderstood him or inadvertently let him down, or because his fear of being emotionally invalidated and re-traumatized caused him to withdraw into a self-protective cocoon to protect his endangered sense of self. At such moments, he either shut me out or verbally attacked me. At one point early in the treatment, Roger got so angry at me that he picked up a chair and threatened to hit me. What kept us going, beside my unflagging commitment to sticking with him in our journey through madness, was Roger's superhuman resolve that his illness would not commandeer his life. As I endured his assaults without retaliation and figured out how I had misunderstood or hurt him and what terror had been triggered, our bond was reestablished and the work resumed.

The safety of our relationship eventually provided an anchor to explore the troubling worlds of his horrendous life—especially the invalidating experiences which drove him crazy, and the "delusions" that were metaphors of traumatic events he had endured but no one had ever understood. Believing that aliens were robbing the encyclopedia he was reading and that rays were being beamed into the bus he was on masterfully evoked the twin experience of being robbed of vital knowledge and taken over by a strange and dangerous outside force that was oblivious to his own wishes and needs.

Over the course of our work together, Roger made profound strides. Understanding the roots and current impact of his delusions helped him gradually develop a fragile faith in the validity of his own reactions. As his self-trust deepened, the voices that ripped him apart lessened. He began feeling more real and alive. He eventually moved into his own apartment, bought a used car that he used to get to work and to our tri-weekly sessions, learned several computer languages, got a job working in a college admissions office, and slowly developed several relationships of value and substance.

My patients—even the most obviously troubled ones—have repeatedly shown me that their words and actions make sense, and that there is a secret goal they are striving for that I must struggle to understand. So, when I hear something that seems self-destructive (like suicidal ideation or self-mutilation), I remember Roger and I try to search for the emotional sanity underneath. It is then easier to find meaning amid the apparent chaos and reach people who are lost and alone and locked into their private worlds of torment and anguish.

Sometimes clarity eludes us. Failure, *as well as understanding*, is part of psychotherapy.

6 Meditating on Failure

"I'd Like to Get to Know You Better"

"We have to end now," I said to Lila, an attractive 30-something woman who was sitting across the room from me on a couch in my office many years ago. I was around the same age. For a moment I looked down, reflecting upon what she had just said about her multiple affairs with various men—the butcher behind the deli counter in the supermarket, the dry cleaner, the local priest. When I looked up a second later, Lila was standing right next to me. My space was crowded. She had a very intense look in her eyes.

"I'd like to get to know you better," she said, turning and pointing to the couch she had just vacated.

Since Lila had just spent the last 50 minutes telling me of her long and tangled history of sexual liaisons, it was obvious that she was asking me to repeat the very behavior that was getting her into trouble.

I was in a no-win situation: Gratify her conscious desires, violate my ethics, spoil the treatment, and emotionally devastate her, or say no to her request and make her feel deeply rejected. Given a "choice" between two lousy options I was reminded of the rabbi and the bird.

There once was a rabbi who was accosted in front of a crowd of people by another rabbi who was jealous of his popularity. The second rabbi issued a challenge: "I have a bird in my hand. Is it alive or is it dead?" The first rabbi knew he was in a pickle. If he said "The bird is alive," the other rabbi would squeeze his hand and crush the bird, and it would die; if he said "The bird is dead," then the second rabbi would open his hand. Not only would the bird fly away, but the first rabbi would lose respect among the villagers. The first rabbi looked at his antagonist and said: "Whether the bird is alive or dead—it seems to me that it is in your hands."

"We have a dilemma," I said to Lila, trying to put her request in *her* hands. "Our time is up. If we act on your desires, we cut off the possibility of understanding what you are feeling and doing. That would be stealing from you. But if we don't do what you want, you may feel that I am cold and withholding and can't help you. What should we do?"

"Talk about it next time," she said as she turned and walked out the door.

DOI: 10.4324/9781003604730-7

Just the answer I was hoping for—or I'd have to fall back on Plan B, which was to politely reject her advances and explore it in the next session.

I'd love to tell you that next week we explored, and shed light on, her conflict, but there was no next session—Lila never came back.

I suspect many therapists would assume that Lila was "resistant to change" and that's what waylaid the treatment. But I wondered then—sometimes even now—if the *therapy* itself was a "failure" and somehow, I let her down. Ending therapy before the work is done, "premature termination" that is not due to physical illness, relocation, or natural disasters, surely doesn't *seem* to qualify as a success. You can't help someone who is not in therapy.

But since I never spoke to Lila again, I can't truly determine what happened and if I failed. Maybe she never returned because I couldn't find a way to constructively respond to her wish to "get to know me better" and she felt rejected, abandoned, or humiliated. Perhaps another therapist with greater empathy, skill, and creativity could have responded differently and she would have returned and worked on what troubled her. Maybe my not "taking the bait" and joining her on the couch made her feel *worse* about someone acting inappropriately in the past who said yes—for example, a relative or religious leader. Or maybe Lila got what she needed—or could handle—at the end of our session and my response helped her see herself in a new and illuminating light. Without more information from Lila, I will never actually know the impact of what I said and did.

Sometimes therapists don't know what is going on—even when the patient is in ongoing treatment. That can be both scary and useful. Scary because the therapist is without a map and a compass; useful because it may aid us in not jumping to premature conclusions about the patient or the course of the treatment. Perhaps for this reason, increasing numbers of contemporary therapists celebrate *not-knowing*.

Western culture has tended to place a premium on all-knowing professionals. We expend tremendous efforts in training and the acquisition of knowledge and expertise which can be wonderfully helpful. *Not knowing* is typically viewed as a *weakness* and a severe limitation. It may signal we are lost and make us feel deficient and inadequate.

However, from a more "Eastern" perspective, thinking we "know" can interfere with direct and intimate contact with life. In Zen Buddhism, for example, not knowing is an opportunity—opening up the possibility of greater richness and depth of experience.

It is written in Chan Buddhist master Hongzhi Zhengjue's (1091–1157) Zen Buddhist classic *The Book of Equanimity* (Wick, 2005) that Hogen had a meeting with his teacher Jizo. Jizo asked him what he had been doing.

"I've been traveling to monasteries and studying with various teachers," Hogen replied.

"What is the point?" Jizo asked.

"I don't know," replied Hogen.

"Not knowing is the most intimate," Jizo said.

This kind of not knowing—being one with what one is doing—listening to the patient without preconceptions can offer an invaluable perspective in the practice of psychotherapy. When a therapist does not know ahead of time what the patient needs, how therapy should unfold or what she will say, she is really listening to the patient, not imposing her own opinion and is therefore less separate and alienated from the client.

All of us need to sit with uncertainty and let go of—or at least hold in abeyance—more of what we "know" so that we can discover what is truly going on.

Accepting uncertainty makes it easier to examine treatments that don't work in a richer light. Failure in psychotherapy is a neglected topic. The cases written about in the psychotherapeutic literature—like most of those in this book—almost always involve people who triumph over obstacles and have happy endings. Therapists rarely write about what doesn't work.

"Try again. Fail again. Fail better," wrote Samuel Beckett in *Worstward Ho* (1983).

Writing about our clinical failures—as well as our successes—could be quite instructive. "One way to approach human error is to see it as a stimulus to the imagination," as Martin Marty (2003, p. 49) recognized. In 1905 Freud initiated what we might call a "literature of failure" in his description of the Dora case, where he maintained that the case was "broken off prematurely" because he "did not succeed in mastering the transference in good time." "The transference," he admitted, "took me unawares" (Freud, 1905, pp. 116–119). Our understanding of clients would be enriched if therapists wrote more about their countertransference, the forces from *their* past and present that catch them unaware and interfere with the treatment.

Drawing on psychoanalyst Arnold Goldberg's helpful taxonomy, we could say that there are cases that: "never get off the ground or never seem to start"; are "interrupted"; "go bad"; "go on and on without obvious improvement"; and "disappoint" (2012, pp. 69–70). The causes include "lack of knowledge" and "lack of empathy" (2012, p. 75).

In a literature of failure, we would reflect on our central assumptions and admit—rather than evade—mistakes. We tend to deny or finesse mistakes or failures in therapy rather than explore them, often blaming them on the patient. While therapy can fail for many reasons ranging from the inexperience of the therapist to the fear of the client to a mismatch between them, many therapists assume that failure comes from the patient. Therapists often speak of the patient's resistance, envy, or self-sabotaging behavior rather than of their own rigidity, fatigue, or lack of imagination. It's easier—and perhaps it feels less demoralizing—to hold patients responsible than to explore our role.

In the last several decades increasing numbers of therapists have examined how whatever happens in therapy—including mistakes or failures—may be shaped more by the interaction of client and therapist than what solely arises inside the mind of the patient. From that perspective therapists can more readily explore how they may have contributed to or even co-created, what doesn't work.

The "supervision" of our patients can be a wonderful resource. When we listen to their reactions to what we say and do as potential commentary or clarification of our work, we allow them to be our teachers and deepen and alter our work together.

Sometimes the reasons for failure are external and explicit: Many years ago, a patient who was beginning to heal a fractured and divided self was blindsided by a drunk driver and died in a car accident before our work was completed. Other times failures are personal—or interpersonal—and more obscure and take digging to excavate.

As I reflect on failures in my practice there have probably been a variety of factors at play. I think I've let certain patients down because I didn't adequately understand what was deeply at stake or I imposed a set theory instead of listening to the person. In other cases, I had an inadequate technique, or my own past conflicts got in the way, or I couldn't build a safe enough bridge to a fearful or self-protective person. I've let patients down because I've talked too little or too much—or was excessively active or too passive.

In recent years I have begun to think of failure in terms of colliding emotional worlds. We each inhabit differently organized universes composed of deep-seated and usually unquestioned values, beliefs, and assumptions. When worlds collide—when you believe that the Me Too and Black Lives Matter movements are forces for cultural healing and your spouse or relative foresees a menace to civilization you (and they) may feel emotionally threatened, unable or unwilling to consider alternative points of view, and try to annihilate or neutralize those you believe threaten you. Hair-trigger reactivity and self-righteous denunciation and censorship often follow.

While a therapist's solitary self-reflection can be helpful to the therapist and the treatment, it is still from the point of view of only one person in the relationship; the therapist. Might client's perspectives offer a window into different aspects of mistakes and failure and even raise new questions about what helps and what hinders therapy?

The only example that I am aware of in the psychotherapeutic literature of cases from both patient and therapist's perspective is the joint diary of a treatment co-authored by Irvin Yalom, an existentially oriented therapist, and Ginny Elkin, a patient of his, entitled *Every Day Gets a Little Closer: A Twice-Told Tale* (1974).

When we meditate on failure and allow our clients to be our supervisors, we might not only *get to know them better* in a way that *enriches* rather than threatens the therapy, but our own clinical work might become immeasurably enriched.

References

Beckett, Samuel. *Worstward Ho*. New York: Grove, 1983.

Freud, Sigmund. "Fragment of an Analysis of a Case of Hysteria." *Standard Edition*, 7:7–122, 1905.

Goldberg, Arnold. *The Analysis of Failure*. New York: Routledge, 2012.

Marty, Martin. "But Even So, Look at That: An Ironic Perspective on Utopias." In *Visions of Utopia*, edited by Edward Rothstein, Herbert Muschamp, and Martin Marty, 49–88. New York: Oxford University Press, 2003.

Wick, Gerry Sishin. *The Book of Equanimity: Illuminating Classic Zen Koans*. Boston: Wisdom Publications, 2005. (Originally written in the 12th century.)

Yalom, Irvin, and Ginny Elkin. *Every Day Gets a Little Closer: A Twice-Told Therapy*. New York: Basic Books, 1974.

7 Curing the Patient of the Illness Created by Their Self-Cure

Healing the Trauma of Neglect in a Zen Buddhist Master

My thoughts, at first aimless, wandered at random, like a greyhound chasing butterflies. As a modicum of focus gradually developed, the noise of mid-Manhattan imperceptibly receded, and attention to inner experience magnified and intensified.

My meditation was interrupted by the shrill sound of the office buzzer.

In the waiting room I encountered a middle-aged man I shall call "Sam." He was tall and gaunt with horn-rimmed glasses, a shaved head, and huge bags under his eyes. We exchanged a firm handshake and solid eye contact.

In my office Sam dove in. He had consulted with me because he felt profoundly alienated and utterly alone. Deeply grounded in both major schools of Zen, indefatigably committed to the truth; open, humble, and sardonic; he was, from all accounts, an immensely talented and maverick Zen teacher who had trained closely with one of the great Buddhist teachers of the twentieth century and embodied what he had learned over several decades of samurai Zen practice.

He had a melancholic and haunted air about him and was riddled with intense anxiety and assaulted by dread. He also described feeling both alien and split in two: a skilled and admired Zen teacher and a scholar and poet and a "screwed up person" who "felt like a reject and a loser." "Forever on the outside looking in," certain that he "didn't belong anywhere," he craved love and felt a deep sense of failure—like a misfit, irremediably disconnected from the human race; longing for normalcy. He claimed he was "playing at living." He admitted he married to have the "semblance of a life" and to "pass for normal with a cover." And he felt invisible. Very invisible. In fact, he called himself "The Invisible Man." I doubt you would even notice him, even if he were standing in your field of vision because he was so self-effacing that he was easy to miss.

In our early sessions, I was immediately struck by how present he was. Nothing seemed to escape his attentive ears and watchful eyes. He listened deeply and was unusually open and disarmingly honest, down-to-earth, without pretense or guile. He displayed a non-defensiveness that many years later still deeply impresses me.

DOI: 10.4324/9781003604730-8

I also admired his self-awareness and his capacity for self-reflection. He had an unusual facility for exploring what he was experiencing, staying directly with a wide range of emotions, and tracking patterns in relationships. I attributed this to his deep meditative practice and his capacity for direct experience more than to his formidable intellect.

In the early sessions I learned that he came by his pessimism, melancholy, and loneliness honestly. Raised by his paternal grandparents, he had little contact with both parents, who were alcoholics. His father showed up occasionally drunk, was completely uninvolved with him, and offered no emotional or concrete assistance. "I hated my father beyond belief," he said.

There was a "conspiracy of silence" about his mother: He was told she was dead. He was also warned "to hang up the phone if a strange woman called." He suspected his mother was alive. He learned from his grandparents that when he was a baby his mother had used his skin as an ashtray and had beaten him with a brine-dipped whip. She left when he was 3.

His paternal grandparents raised him on the outskirts of a metropolitan area on the West Coast. He led an intensely solitary childhood. His grandfather was private and hidden, an outwardly rational man who became a Christian scientist and secretly hoarded Jehovah's Witness *Watchtower* magazines and spent most of his time in his basement workshop, crafting hundreds of miniature sailing ships in bottles.

His grandmother was senile toward the end of his childhood and seemed superstitious and irrational. "She spent most of her time lying in bed among her large collection of dolls, wearing layers of house dresses she hardly took off and her Dodgers baseball cap." When a friend of Sam's came over to their house, they jubilantly served strawberry ice cream on a block of frozen French fries.

His grandparents "hated each other, and hardly ever spoke." The resounding abandonments and emotional neglect were "devastating." Sam became ashamed and intolerant of his own needs. This led to massive self-deprivation. He convinced himself that going to college was "selfish." He only applied to one college and thought he'd skip university, live with his grandparents, and be a typist and write poetry.

He assumed he "must have somehow been worthless to the core." But he couldn't figure out what he had done wrong. The shadow of essential badness and inadequacy stayed with him throughout his life; it was never touched or transformed despite decades of intensive and wholehearted Zen training and practice, leaving him feeling bereft and angry.

Sam drew great solace from languages and ideas. He devoted his considerable talents to scholastic pursuits and athletics and graduated first in his high school class at 16.

"If you leave this house, it will kill me," his grandmother said. He applied to an Ivy League college, but never heard from it. Several months after the college acceptances were sent, he reached high up into the back of a cabinet for a cup and discovered an envelope. He pulled it out and noticed it was addressed to him. He opened it and learned that he had received a complete scholarship. He felt his grandparents had betrayed him by hiding his acceptance letter.

"Childhood led to extreme alienation," he told me. "I was never touched or reached. And I was filled with alienation and despair; the despair of never having a fulfilling life."

After a stellar academic performance in the first year of college, he found out his mother was alive. "Would you like to meet your mother?" his inebriated father asked him over the phone. Sam was disturbed and angry but agreed to go.

When he met his mother, she was drunk, which only deepened his revulsion. She told him he was better off without her. He left after she downed a row of sloe gin fizzes.

He was 17. And shattered.

The drunken meeting, the way he had been betrayed about his mother's supposed death, and his abandonment by both parents induced a homicidal rage. He moved to Europe for a year, unable to speak and express the condition he was in, in his words, "catatonic."

Upon his return to America, he graduated with high honors from college at 20 and was accepted into a doctoral program in literature. He read all the literature on metaphor in English, French, and German—including Max Black's *Language and Philosophy* and Jacques Derrida's "White Magic," Ernst Cassirer's *Symbolic Forms*, and Suzanne Langer's *Philosophy in a New Key*. When his doctoral advisor relocated, he told Sam to contact him in two weeks, after he settled into his new home. When Sam called, the advisor acted like they had never met and dumped him—another abandonment.

Immersion in Zen

In his 20s, a friend introduced Sam to Zen. He took to it immediately. He read no Zen literature, not wanting to intellectualize or contaminate the process, and just meditated. At his first meditation retreat the teacher, Eido Roshi, told Sam, "Kill the watcher." "Die on the cushion and you'll never have to die again." Sam found this easy and natural, in part because it tragically replicated the annihilation of his being he had experienced with his parents and grandparents. Sam quit his newly acquired tenured professorship and became a full-time student of Zen.

At his first retreat he reached *kensho*—he had an enlightenment experience when he felt one with everything. The boundaries between inner and outer evaporated and he saw to the depths of and through his constructed sense of self. "I felt as if something like an earthquake or an implosion was about to happen," he wrote in his unpublished autobiography. "Everything around me looked exceedingly odd, as if the glue separating things had started to melt. By the time I got to my room I was weightless; there was no gravity. Then the earthquake or implosion, body and mind dropping off, occurred.

There was an incredible explosion of light coming from inside and outside simultaneously, and everything disappeared into that light . . . there was no longer a here versus there, a this versus that . . . I understood nothing except that nothing would ever seem the same to me . . . And despite the fact that I had no understanding whatever of what had happened (nor do I now), this experience changed my life completely."

His meditative practice and his insights continued to expand and ripen during his studies with Zen masters from several different traditions.

He taught a course on Buddhism. An older Japanese man sat in the front row all semester listening intently without saying a word. After the last class, the man came up to Sam and invited him to tea. As Sam and Maezumi Roshi, the head of the Los Angeles Zen Center, drank sake together Maezumi told Sam he was a Zen master and wanted Sam to be his dharma heir, a rare honor in which a student is chosen by their teacher to eventually be a successor. "Forget about it," Sam said, "you're drunk."

Sam studied with Maezumi's protégé and was eventually chosen to be one of his successors. Sam also received an informal transmission from Soen Nakagawa, a Roshi many consider the greatest Zen master of the twentieth century, who told him he had had an enlightenment experience at his first retreat. Despite the fact that Sam was a Zen prodigy, he couldn't answer the question one of his teachers asked that he sensed was central to his being: "What is it you *want*?"

"The question renders me dumbfounded," he said.

How could he know when he had been brutally abused and neglected?

Further relationships with several Zen masters increased Sam's alienation. He left several he was slated to succeed when his teachers became embroiled in sexual or financial scandals. Whereas most of the students turned a blind eye to the way these men exploited female students sexually or used members of the community to build a spiritual empire, Sam refused to compromise his principles in order to keep his standing with the teachers and in the community. He exposed and left each teacher, even though he was slated to be a successor. This undermined his position and visibility in the rather cliquey American Zen community. He became again, an outcast; a Zen-master-without-a-temple. And, a man without a home. He reported, at the time, "I have no place to go. Returning to the real world," he added, "was not a world to me."

His father died several years later: They never reconciled, and he was "guilty over hating him so much." He had a "profound sense of nowhere to go" and that "nothing mattered."

And then his wife betrayed him. When he found her in bed with another man it merely confirmed his deep-seated belief that he was worthless and there was no place on earth for him. In psychoanalysis he realized he had never really been seen or emotionally touched by his wife.

Sam supported himself by leading meditation retreats and teaching literature and Zen in various colleges and universities. His students loved him, but he remained on the fringes of the Zen mainstream, as former disciples moved up the American Zen Buddhist ranks and garnered positions and teaching opportunities he rightfully deserved.

At the beginning of treatment Sam appeared vulnerable and terrified, tense and fragile. The source of his fear was not immediately apparent. Later we recognized that beneath the fear was shame. The origins of that humiliation took some time to emerge.

Several months into the treatment, I learned that before Sam began psychotherapy with me, he had been staying at an inn across the street from a Zen monastery. Years earlier, he had spent the night at the same inn after his marriage ceremony at the Zen center. Sam asked the Roshi who ran the monastery, a man who credited Sam with inspiring his meditation practice, if he could live there and do intensive practice. The teacher said no. Sam was angry. Staying at the inn and being disconnected from the Zen center reminded him of his separation from his wife and his frustrated Zen path and was disturbing and disorienting. He felt rebuffed again in trying to find a place for himself.

In a shame-filled phone message Sam left for me he said he had the fantasy of exposing himself, of standing on the inn's front porch and opening his robe. He called himself "weak and cowardly" for revealing this over the phone. A few weeks later in an actual session he admitted he had acted on this fantasy, and that was, in fact, the reason he initiated treatment.

He feared I would judge him and shame him. He was also terrified he would be sent to jail and his life would be over. When he talked about the incident, he had a very concrete opinion of what he had done. He viewed it and judged it very literally. It was sick, he said, and perverted, and he was "bad." I knew he was a kind and empathic man and not a danger to anyone. I tried to interest him in exploring the meaning of what he did. What did he feel before, during, and after he exposed himself and what was he trying to communicate? In other words, what was the action *saying*?

Breaking Out of the Prison of Invisibility

After we had explored various possible meanings and functions, I said, "I wonder if you exposed yourself because you were desperately trying to break through the horrific prison of invisibility, the wall of alienation between you and the rest of the world, so you could finally be seen."

"I am so glad you said that," he replied. He looked deeply relieved and moved. I could sense his trust in me growing. I later learned that when I said this he felt truly "seen" for the first time. He noticeably relaxed, and the dread left his face and body. "It was a plea for help. I feel like I'm from a different planet . . . a weird mystic."

Our sessions over the next six months had a remarkable openness and intimacy. We engaged in a transparent, no-holds-barred dialogue with minimum defensiveness and maximum honesty. An unusual fondness and respect developed between Sam and me. The therapeutic relationship—and the treatment—expanded. Themes of abandonment and neglect, passivity and invisibility took center stage. We got clearer about how his parents, his doctoral advisor, and some of his Zen teachers abandoned him, and how he neglected himself personally and professionally.

We both realized that Dogen's "Genjokoan" or "The Way of Everyday Life," a seminal and often quoted thirteenth-century Zen text (1233/2002), resonated with how Sam felt:

To study the Buddha Way is to study the self.
To study the self is to forget the self.
To forget the self is to be enlightened by the 10,000 dharmas.

On a profound emotional level, Dogen's famous words perfectly captured Sam's neglect by his family of origin. This Zen text mirrored Sam's experience of himself and his view of the world when he realized, midway through psychoanalysis, that many people in his life (from his mother and father to his graduate advisor and a Zen teacher) had forgotten about him.

"Forgetting the self," in Zen, refers to letting go of the pervasive, taken-for-granted, and silently debilitating, self-referential self-consciousness that alienates most of us in Western culture from each other and ourselves. Sam's highly developed capacity, in this sense, to "forget" himself and forego such self-consciousness aided him in being deeply engaged and manifesting an unusual presence. I am certain it helped him access his buried history of trauma in psychoanalysis and explore a wide range of emotions with little judgment and great depth.

But in ordinary parlance outside of Zen circles, "forget oneself" has, of course, a more harmful connotation: It can mean to neglect ourselves; to fall asleep to ourselves; to disregard who we are and our wishes and needs. Sam, unfortunately, also experienced this kind of self-forgetfulness. And the consequences were disastrous.

Sam's strategy to protect himself against further re-traumatization, what psychoanalyst Masud Khan in The *Privacy of the Self* called his "practice of self-cure" (1974, p. 97), was to forget about and abandon himself. If there was no self, then there was no one who had been forsaken. Sam was self-neglectful, inadvertently repeating what had traumatized him in his youth. He didn't need his mother, father, wife, academic advisor, or Zen teacher to dump him; Sam beat them to the punch. He was an incredible survivor, but deeply passive. While he felt "invisible" and longed to be "seen," he dismissed his feelings and his needs, "feasting on crumbs" and settling for emotional deprivation while using meditation to more wholeheartedly engage whatever else he was experiencing.

Sam was very skilled at being-intimate-with-this-moment, appreciating everything from the birds serenading him in the early morning outside his window to the taste of a cup of tea, yet he unwittingly deprived himself of much human contact, fulfillment, and joy.

The psychotherapist's own willingness to examine their assumptions and biases, especially those that may interfere with understanding the patient, is crucial to the success of therapy, as I suggested in Chapter 6. Ever since Freud, psychotherapists have known they can interfere with the progress of psychotherapy. Such countertransference, the therapist's characteristic ways of organizing their experience and responding to the patient, could be viewed as the therapist's contribution to obstacles in the treatment.

Sam and I worked our way through a countertransferential knot, what one might think of as addressing moments of failure, and that intensified our work and aided Sam in transforming his self-deprivation. As Sam's trust in me grew, his massive unmet dependency needs emerged. He became very passive and needy, adopting a stance of pseudo-incompetence regarding self-care and navigating the world. He acted like he could not manage any of the practical aspects of his life and other people were responsible for taking care of him. Like many neglected people, his (self-)deprivation became intolerable and morphed into entitlement, as psychoanalyst Peter Shabad aptly noted in *Despair and the Return of Hope* (2007). *In other words, the world frustrated me, now you owe me.* I was supposed to make up for what Sam never received from his parents or grandparents.

At first, I approached what Jody Davies and Mary Frawley in *Treating the Adult Survivor of Sexual Abuse* (1994), call the "entitled child demanding rescue," by trying to be empathic and attuned to his neglect. But his neediness and sense of entitlement expanded. Repressed wishes for emotional nurturance he never received became needs that I and other people must fulfill now. I subtly constrained myself by trying to override my irritation about his entitlement, rather than studying it. Striving to be empathic and responsive trumped understanding the source of his emotional hunger and his self-damaging response to it. I reacted to my irritation, which had perhaps shifted, at times into low-level anger, by slightly withdrawing from him when he was highly needy.

Preserving the Pain

We eventually explored this pattern. At first, we discussed it gingerly. He was afraid of being abandoned by me. As I responded without defensiveness to his muted irritation, he elaborated. His pseudo-incompetent, passive stance—a "going on strike"—was designed to preserve a snapshot of his unwitnessed pain and keep alive the hope other people could witness what had been done to him so that someone might save him and be the mother he never had.

As I understood this on an emotional level, and he felt seen and heard, he no longer needed to embrace his symptom as a way of preserving a snapshot of his unwitnessed emotional pain. And this enabled him to begin taking more responsibility for his own life.

Several months later he didn't show up for three weeks because of sickness and snowstorms. In between he called and we had phone sessions. At the beginning of the third phone session, he said, "Please don't abandon me."

The irony hit me like a gale-force wind. "I'm staring at my empty couch," I gently but firmly said, "*You* are the one doing the abandoning . . . Are you abandoning yourself the way you have always been abandoned?"

"I never thought about it that way," he said. "I think there is something profoundly disturbing and true about that."

He went through a phase of fear and depression. Depression as he awakened to what he had done to himself; fear that he would never get beyond self-neglect.

"I got frightened that for ages I had abandoned my life," he said. "I realized my response to being abandoned was to abandon myself and neglect myself. From psychoanalysis I'm learning that the shadow side of Buddhism is the notion of no-self, which can lead to self-abandonment and self-neglect." He believed this aspect of psychoanalysis was consistent with Zen master Bodhidharma's interpretation of the precept of not killing as "not nursing a view of extinction," not trying to eliminate aspects of our humanness, realizing that at best we integrate and come to terms with, rather than get rid of troubling experiences.

Sam then began talking about how his analysis had touched on core issues and feelings that decades of intense and sincere meditation practice missed, like his abuse and neglect and self-depriving behavior. He began taking himself more seriously and being less self-neglectful. He sought out companionship and became less isolated. He also focused on constructing a life that reflected his current passions and interests.

He now wanted a life, felt entitled to one, and was taking steps for that to happen. "I have fantasies about having a relationship and even sex." And he became more available for each. I learned when he was younger, he enjoyed socializing but had fallen into a harmful habit of self-protective isolation. He moved closer to the Zen community he had founded, where he had been a non-resident teacher. He not only appeared more buoyant and less melancholic, but he was also more visible, less isolated, and more engaged. He was eager to make his life his own.

Toward the end of treatment, Sam said: "It is a source of great pathos to reflect that without psychoanalysis I might have died without having been reunited with myself! And in that sense, without having truly lived. I don't feel divided anymore," he added, "and I finally know what I want: To be at ease within my own skin." He felt "joy," he said, the joy, I suspect, of a man who was on the road to living a life he could honestly call his own.

References

Davies, Jody Messler, and Mary Gail Frawley. *Treating the Adult Survivor of Childhood Sexual Abuse: A Psychoanalytic Perspective*. New York: Basic Books, 1994.
Dogen, "Genjokoan" or "The Way of Everyday Life." In *On Zen Practice: Body, Breath, and Mind*, edited by Taizen Maezumi & Bernie Glassman, 133–138. Boston: Wisdom Publications, 2002. (Originally written 1233)
Khan, Masud. *The Privacy of the Self*. New York: International Universities Press, 1974.
Shabad, Peter C. *Despair and the Return of Hope: Echoes of Mourning in Psychotherapy*. Lanham: Jason Aronson, 2007.

8 The Reluctant Sensei
Zen and Self-Healing

One of the ironies of psychoanalysis is that the most personal of disciplines is often written about impersonally; the therapist—and the patient's experience of their therapist and the therapy—is left out. While this is slowly changing—there are more examples of this in the therapeutic literature—the emotional distance of the therapist still pervades the field of mental health.

After I finished a draft of the previous chapter, I shared it with Sam.

"I like it a lot—it was an accurate portrayal of our work together," he said a few days later.

I sensed a reservation. "Do I hear a 'but'?" I asked.

"I really liked it," he said, his voice not convincing me.

"Stay with—and take seriously—your mixed feelings."

"In preserving my confidentiality, the chapter ironically may have repeated my invisibility," he replied.

After we explored what he meant by this, I asked Sam if he wanted to write about his experience of therapy. He didn't, but he had several suggestions. "You could further undo my invisibility by calling me by my true name—Lou Mitsunen Nordstrom—and indicating that I am a philosophy professor on the East Coast instead of a literature professor on the West Coast. And you could write about my influence on you."

I decided to try.

In the process of our work together, something magical happened—Mitsunen (which means "now mind") became my teacher.

I began studying Zen with Mitsunen from the onset of therapy because we both felt it would be immensely helpful for me to have a more intimate sense of what was the center of his life. My previous two decades plus immersion in Buddhism had been in Theravadin Buddhism and Vipassana meditation—the original teachings and practice of the historical Buddha. I had read Zen texts but never formally studied Zen. I attended a lecture by one of Mitsunen's teachers in the late 1970s, but didn't feel moved to study with him. Had I, I would have soon come in contact with Mitsunen, his successor, and chief disciple.

For the reader to understand Mitsunen's influence on my life I need to say more about myself and my studies with him.

DOI: 10.4324/9781003604730-9

I too have felt for much of my life like an Invisible Man; essentially unseen and unappreciated; fitting uneasily into the worlds I grew up in and later inhabited. Each world—my family, Buddhism, psychoanalysis—always felt too focused on an exclusive and exclusionary identity and an allegiance to a narrow set of principles that were inimical to freedom and creativity. In addition, I often felt my abilities were unrecognized and there was a huge gap between how I was viewed by other people and what I actually offered.

Many years ago, Robert Stolorow, a psychoanalyst I greatly admired for his enormous—and original—contribution to psychoanalytic thinking, said to the audience at a conference: "My assumption is that no one ever listens to me."

I have a similar expectation. The eldest of two siblings, much of my earlier life was devoted to rescuing—and not threatening—my troubled younger brother; a damaged soul, who has spent much of his adult life not being a model citizen. While the cause and purpose of his behavior baffled everyone, what is clear to me now is that he didn't receive what he sorely needed—love, connection, esteem—and has spent a lifetime seeking something he has never found.

My parents, who seemed overwhelmed and shamed, recruited me to save him. An atheist, my mother created an Eleventh Commandment for me alone: "Put the other first and disregard yourself." Loyal to a fault, I accommodated her wishes by ignoring how I felt, minimizing my academic and athletic triumphs so as not to make my brother feel envious or diminished, and denying my own right to a life. I felt it was my job to "heal wounded sparrows." I gravitated toward people with severe emotional conflicts and too many of my relationships involved a one-sided caretaking that left me feeling neglected and deprived. This included several dates with women with physical handicaps simply because I felt sorry for them.

I have often felt alone, invisible, homeless. In a tragic Faustian bargain, I "get" a home by fitting in wherever I find myself and giving myself up. I became pathologically accommodating to the needs of my parents and brother to the exclusion of my own as Brandchaft described in *Toward an Emancipatory Psychoanalysis* (2010). *I remained quiet or silent in the face of crazy behavior on their part.*

I became so adept at hiding my interests and talents and organizing my relationships with other people so as to leave myself out, that I was taken for granted by other people, as well as myself, and buried alive. And I didn't even know it. I only later realized that I had several one-sided "friendships" with highly narcissistic people.

Eventually, I joined the family view of me as a rube, or a patsy—even after I graduated from two Ivy League schools and was a college-level athlete—because my brother had vastly superior entrepreneurial talents and was a "better earner" than I. My parents never seemed to notice that he applied his talents to shady enterprises such as white-collar crimes.

Unfortunately, not only did my parents and brother and I speak incompatible languages, but we also inhabited diametrically opposed worlds. And there was neither a recognition of nor a place for me in my home. My parents never asked me about what it was like growing up with a psychopathic brother. And my mother demanded that I join her denial of my brother's illness and blame bigoted and persecutory authorities—or my accomplishments—for his travails.

My emotional splint—the way I tried to heal myself by myself (which became a self-created prison)—was accommodating to the madness that was my family, being hyper-mindful of the other (which has been an asset as a psychoanalyst), and putting myself in "lockdown" and minimizing and hiding my value so as to not threaten my brother. This self-protective strategy prevented me from being blind-sided and re-traumatized by my mother's annihilating invalidation of my being. It also kept alive the hope that the respect and recognition that had forever been absent from my parents might be forthcoming. But it caused me to not take seriously my own feelings and needs.

Because I was not listened to—or seen—in my family of origin, it's not surprising to me that for many years I didn't really see, or trust, my own value. I knew that to liberate myself from the prison I had unwittingly created in order to protect myself I had to see myself accurately, take seriously my own feelings, and relate to other people less self-deprecatingly. Only then could I have a life of my own and be myself.

After a great deal of progress working on the trauma of invisibility in my own therapy, a prerequisite of my training to be a therapist, I still felt, in certain vital ways, like I was living inside the prison I had created to try to minimize the ordeal of my childhood. I still lived a diminished life, minimized my feelings, and neglected my value. The liberator of other imprisoned souls was incarcerated himself.

Zen and Self-Healing

In an unexpected turn, the Zen master himself was of inestimable help in freeing me from the confines of the cell I had erected in order to survive.

There's a Zen of everything in the new millennium: art and business, leadership and cooking. And yet, there's not a lot of actual Zen.

Zen is simple. Direct. Unadorned. Un-self-conscious intimacy with this moment. Zen is about being a real human being and showing up for life. And playing the hand you are dealt wholeheartedly. Mitsunen taught me this. And he embodied it.

Mitsunen was a real human being—warm and approachable—who brought a refreshing transparency to the teacher–student relationship. Nothing was off limits and anything we thought or felt—from the wisdom and folly of Zen or ourselves—was fair game. This fostered an intimacy between us that was rare. Since we related without pretense or guile, we both saw each other as we actually were.

Mitsunen never tried to bolster himself at my expense. Instead, he affirmed me. When I questioned Zen principles or practices, he was completely receptive to what I said. He let me teach him—and find my own path. When I sheepishly told him that my own practice of meditation integrated two different methods —Vipassana, or insight meditation, and Zen breath counting—and therefore wasn't strictly Zen, he said he knew that from things I had previously told him and he was more interested in my finding my own path and teaching in my own way, than being a clone of him. I don't assume this always goes on between people in power like spiritual teachers and their subordinates, and analytic supervisors and their supervisees—and I don't take it for granted.

In my Zen studies with him we twice explored koans, those elusive questions Zen teachers ask their students that defy rational explanation and liberate an un-self-conscious, intimate relationship to life. The first time we did koan study we proceeded in a traditional way. Faced with a question, for example, "How do you take the next step on the top of a hundred-foot pole?" I tried to demonstrate that I understood and could embody my answer.

"You have a genuine facility for this," he said, as I quickly moved through koan study. Nonetheless, I still hid my value and seduced other people into perpetuating my invisibility. For example, I had several completed manuscripts that I shared with practically no one. And only a reluctant sensei would not tell hardly anyone he had himself become a Zen teacher.

Highly attuned and masterful at intuiting a student's needs, Mitsunen was an iconoclastic teacher—a Zen jazz improviser—who used any tool at his disposal in his search to help me. He suggested a second round of koan study. But we took a less traditional tack geared, I now realize, not only to deconstruct my conditioning, but to facilitate a break-through in my self-understanding and behavior.

Spiritual students are among the most competitive people on the planet. In their hunger for advancement, they are often spiritual chameleons—feeding the teacher what they imagine they want to garner favor so that they can impress the teacher and become a teacher or have power over other students in the spiritual organization.

Because I was allergic to the supplication that passes for devotion that spiritual students often employ to get their teacher's approval and advance up the hierarchy of the spiritual organization—I suspect it reminded me of my brother's self-serving dishonesty—Mitsunen confronted me with an opposite dilemma. "You're a life-long student and now it's time to be a teacher," he often said to me. After the warm glow of his compliment faded, I remained a dutiful apprentice—thereby maintaining what I only now realize was my perverted loyalty to my damaged brother. I often acted like a student, not a teacher—deferring to less experienced colleagues and ascribing to them an authority and an expertise that they didn't deserve.

The second time we did koan study Mitsunen—probably cognizant of my tendency to hide and not claim my talents—recommended an unconventional, and for me, inspired method of study. "Zen teachers and students have a knee-jerk veneration of koans," he said. "You are correct that we often attribute to tradition an automatic and unearned authority that neglects the need for innovation in the present. Your intuition that some koans are dated and neglect emotions is also true," he said. "Trust your reactions as you read various koans and allow that to shape which ones you delve into."

What was most enlightening was not this approach to koan study, which was valuable, but the spirit of self-trust—faith in myself—that it cultivated, that carried over into the rest of my life. I began relating to life more directly and intuitively; trusting what I felt, as opposed to automatically accommodating other people's wishes and needs.

While as a psychoanalyst I know that emotions often deceive and mislead, as well as signal what we value and fear; Mitsunen's simple-seeming suggestion—which in effect forced me to be my own teacher—demonstrated a powerful faith in me, and was a creative way of helping me trust my experience on a more intimate level. And that immeasurably aided me in appreciating my value, which eventually liberated me from the prison house of hiding who I really am.

An adult client once described standing outside a ballroom. Inside there was a professional conference involving the most talented colleagues in her field. While she had the credentials and accomplishments to be on the stage participating in the conference, she had never been asked. As hundreds of people walked past her into the ballroom, no one even noticed her. She felt like she didn't even exist.

Imagining I am her helps me describe Mitsunen's impact on my life. Not only was he the lone person who stopped to speak to me, but he lovingly chided me for not being on the stage where I belonged.

"You are already in the ballroom," he said. "You just don't realize it. You suffer from what I call a pathological Bodhisattva complex—putting the other ahead of the self. You act like a student, but you are already a teacher. It's time to embrace that."

In our next meeting, several days later I shared an epiphany: "I am already 'teaching' Zen, I am just doing it practicing psychoanalysis."

"Not just," he smiled. "You are looking to be a teacher, and you are already teaching," he replied. "You are already there—without anything else happening like a formal Zen ceremony—but you don't realize it . . . Doing therapy you are already a Zen teacher. That is your Zen."

Mitsunen built my confidence—helping me inhabit, instead of sleepwalking through, my life—which aided me in believing in, and being, myself. Seen by him, I saw myself and began trusting my voice, which made it easier to fully be myself and take my rightful place in the world. This took various forms—from seeking more reciprocal relationships with other people, to jettisoning narcissistic colleagues, to devoting more time and attention to what I am passionate about, to cultivating my own style of teaching, combining meditation practice, talks integrating meditation and psychotherapy, and spontaneous dialogues with the audience. Some years ago, the director of a Buddhist center asked me to teach the Buddhist-teachers-in-training the way I listen and respond to students.

"Say 'Sensei' three times when you awake," Mitsunen suggested after he named me a dharma heir, a Zen teacher (-in-training). Mostly I do, sometimes I forget. But even when I don't remember to, I finally see myself as a "Zen guy." And that has changed my life. I am not only referring to the fact that I taught at Buddhist centers, have worked in psychotherapy with several Buddhist teachers, and relate to the world more wholeheartedly and un-self-consciously. I have also regained the innocence and passion that was put in cold storage when I was a young man.

"Thank you for being alive," Mitsunen often said to me as he was leaving our sessions.

Only rare people hit bullseyes on a target that others don't even see. "Thank *you* for being alive," I replied.

Reference

Brandchaft, Bernard, Shelley Doctors, and Dorienne Sorter. *Toward an Emancipatory Psychoanalysis: Brandchaft's Intersubjective Vision*. New York: Routledge, 2010.

9 Memorials of Our Unwitnessed Pain

Suicide is a Lonely Affair

For years, Lawrence, an emotionally deprived, but materially pampered, young adult, had spoken of suicide. A superior student with several friends and varied interests, he was struggling with the anger he felt toward his intrusive, emotionally troubled mother, who had been in and out of mental health facilities during his adolescence. Although the anger rarely surfaced, Lawrence was a hostage to its presence and its hold on him. He also felt betrayed by his passive father, who, while overindulging him, failed to protect him from his mother. Lawrence never spoke openly of not feeling protected, but his contempt toward his father spoke volumes. Outrage against political injustices and an extreme identification with victims of oppression were the channels for his deprivation and anger. He maintained an outward persona grown on the thin soil of a dilettante's encounter with Eastern thought. And although he spoke of empathy toward political prisoners, it seemed superficial and impersonal. His readings of popular, watered-down versions of Asian thought, which he only half digested, didn't include the practices they recommended. He signed the letters he showed me, "Being peace."

Peace and self-acceptance were the last things he radiated. A burning anger, arrogance, and emotional detachment were more like it. When the pressure built up and Lawrence's anger outflanked his stance of "being peace," the knives came out and his wrist or forearm was faintly carved, actually etched, not enough to hurt him, but just enough so everyone would panic and finally pay attention to him. The thin, shallow scars on his arm were tangible signs of the pain he could not put into words.

The mere threat of his self-cutting was enough to send his parents scurrying for the psychiatrists and the meds. No shrinking violet, Lawrence had everyone convinced that he was an emotionally fragile, imminently suicidal risk. I wondered if holding his parents (and therapists) hostage was a way of evening the score for the emotional torture his parents had inflicted on him.

I was the latest in a long line of therapists he had seen. Not worked with but *seen*. For Lawrence didn't really ever work on himself. He showed up, resisted efforts to make the situation better, and when he had had enough, which happened periodically, he pulled out the knives and went to work—on

DOI: 10.4324/9781003604730-10

his arms. He gave me the impression that he liked the power to punish. I wondered if it was the only place where he felt he could make an impact, where he wasn't powerless.

In my office many years ago, Lawrence spoke of feeling suicidal. I don't remember the specific precipitating event for this latest threat, but we talked around it for a while as he evaded my attempts to understand how he felt. We had been here before and I realized that he was invested in staying exactly where he was.

On this particular afternoon, a loud ringing interrupted the session. He looked at me. "It might be a fire alarm," I said. "We may need to evacuate the building. Let me go out and check."

The noise was coming from the direction of the radio in my waiting room. I fiddled with several buttons until I figured out how to turn off the alarm that someone had turned on.

When I returned to my office Lawrence said with some fear: "We'd better leave the building."

From the urgency in his voice I could tell that his concern for his physical well-being was sincere and that he was anxious to get out of my office as fast as possible. This made no sense if he really wanted to die.

"Why should we leave the building?" I asked.

"Because we might be in danger," he said, his voice betraying a hint of panic.

"But you want to die, so why do you care?"

Lawrence stared at me, speechless—an actor whose script was suddenly blank.

"Suicide is a lonely affair," I said, "I can't imagine anything worse than dying alone, so I'll stay here with you in your last moments on earth."

"I don't want to *die*," Lawrence said emphatically. His face suddenly had color. His declaration had broken through the protective facade of suicidal posturing.

Most of us don't want to die, but many of us may be ambivalent about resolving our problems and living a better life. Although not resolving them undoubtedly causes us pain, we may also gain a secret benefit—providing on-going snapshots and "memorials" of our un-witnessed pain so that we can attempt to communicate with a loved one who can't hear our silent screams. We may also lessen the pressure on ourselves to succeed; excuse away failures; and punish those who have wronged us. Holding onto our problems keeps alive the hope of getting emotional validation and love that we sorely missed. It is a "self-cure" for the "illness" of being unloved.

Therapy is not poker, and I wouldn't recommend bluffing as a regular technique, but when the opportunity presented itself to test Lawrence's wish to die—a claim he clung to for dear life—I seized it to help him see that it was a charade. He still mentioned suicide a few times after that, but it had no more heat. When he stopped acting like he was committed to dying, he began focusing on living—pursuing his passions and dreams.

It's been several years since I saw Lawrence, but I heard from his father several months ago. He wrote: "Hope this finds you well. Wanted you to know that my son is doing much better. He's no angel—he and my wife still go at it in a way that disturbs me—but he no longer holds us hostage with threats of suicide. And he got a master's degree in English literature and is teaching English and studying Aikido in Japan."

A patient of mine once said that "suicide is inverted homicide." The founder of Aikido, Morihei Ueshiba (2002) described his art as the "Way of Harmony." I found it intriguing that my former patient was now studying a martial art whose purpose was to end all violence and bring peace into the world. I wondered if this meant that he was going beyond the place our work had left him—choosing living over a diminished existence in which he held others (and himself) hostage.

The American Foundation for Suicide Prevention (AFSP) informs us that in 2022 suicide was the 11th leading cause of death in the US and 49,476 Americans died by suicide that year. No two people with suicidal thoughts or fantasies are completely alike. Some can't stomach the indignities of a terminal illness or a life without a loved one. Others are haunted by unbearable grief or anger or shame for a career or relationship failure or for not fulfilling the expectations of other people or themselves. Still others wish to punish someone or escape from horrific circumstances like political torture, rape, or a natural disaster. And then there are those people who have lost interest in life.

The wish to "end it all" can be a way to kill, silence, or escape from psychic, physical, or spiritual pain. Hopelessness. Humiliation. Betrayal. Terror. Despair. Since it doesn't seem possible to find a way through the agony, killing off despised parts of oneself and escaping the unbearable torment feels like the only viable option, even if it means sacrificing the rest of ourselves.

There is little margin for error with suicidal people. I remember a time some years ago when I was treating four suicidal patients at the same time. I was on hyper-alert, treading water in the deep end, with very little in reserve, knowing that everything rested on quickly and deeply understanding each client's unique torment. Often the person's wish to die was like a gale force wind—if you weren't careful, it could blow you over.

Discussions of youth suicide aptly note the different warning signs such as feelings of sadness or hopelessness, declining school performance, loss of pleasure/interest in social and sports activities, sleeping too little or too much, changes in weight and appetite.

When is suicide an imminent risk? And what guides the clinician in assessing danger? I attend to both the person's condition and their relationship to other people and to me. I might ask how they picture the funeral and how life goes on after the suicide. How does the person considering suicide imagine the survivors will react? Who will show up for the funeral? Who will care? I listen to both what the person consciously says and what their voice and body indirectly communicate. Is there sadness? Hopelessness? Despair? How much bitterness and spitefulness is there? Does the person want to exact revenge against someone else? Are there any constructive outlets for the person's feelings? Is there any connection to other people or to me? How comfortable is the suicidal person with relying on other people and asking for help? The greater the isolation the higher the risk. The dangers increase if the person has lost connection with other people, refuses to seek help, is getting their affairs in order and increasingly checking out of life.

The greatest risk for suicide is often when the person begins to feel slightly better. In the depth of depression, one may feel so paralyzed that most actions—even self-destructive ones—feel too overwhelming.

The only thing that gave me solace when I was treating several suicidal people at once was the recognition, which came and went, that I wasn't responsible for their lives, but for fully engaging our work. Sometimes this offered slight relief from the terrible pressure I felt, but often the weight of responsibility overrode it.

The Association for Suicide Prevention suggests three things parents and other teens can do when dealing with a child or peer who is very depressed. Parents can get their child medical or psychological help, support the child, and become informed themselves. Friends or classmates of a troubled teen can take their friend's actions seriously, talk to a trusted adult about their concerns, and encourage their friend to seek professional help.

But the best protection in my experience is a life of meaning. Cicero, like Plato, said that philosophizing is nothing other than getting ready to die. I side with Montaigne, who believed that learning how to live will help us live—and die—in peace: "If we have known how to live steadfastly and calmly we shall know how to die the same way . . . death is indeed the ending of life, but not therefore its end: it puts an end to it but it is not its objective."

Several suicidal young adults I have treated over the years have taught me that their main problem was not the wish to die. That was just the overt *symptom*. The real problem was that each of them had a profound lack of meaning in their lives. This occurred because they were so busy accommodating to what other people wanted—parents' goals for them and/or peer group pressure to be a certain way—rather than learning about and pursuing what they wanted or needed. They gradually lost touch with—or never even developed—their own passions or dreams. As a result, they were literally living lives that were empty and not their own. For such people the answer to the question, "Whose Life Is It Anyway?" is a resounding "Not Mine."

After listening to Adam, a depressed teenager, describe in a desultory manner, for nearly the entire session, the way he strove to comply with his parents' wishes and never disappoint them, and how guilty he felt for minor transgressions, I asked him if he had ever felt suicidal. He was shocked.

"What made you ask me that?" Adam said.

"If *my* life was not my own, I wouldn't want to keep living it," I replied.

His shoulders dropped. His relief at being "found" in the wilderness of his private despair changed his entire body language.

Although Adam had never expressed thoughts of suicide, he was quietly checking out of life. This was reflected in his cutting school, staying holed up in his room for hours at a time and taking little joy in living the life others had planned for him. And while he did not really want to die, he was despairing about how to live with any kind of passion and joy. As we examined his life, what emerged was that his relationship with his parents was filled with conformity and fear. In devoting all his energies to keeping the peace between his hypercritical mother and depressed and detached father, he had ignored fundamental questions about who he was and how he wanted to live. His creativity was hidden and buried beneath his attempts to please his parents and ensure that they didn't fight or get divorced on his account.

"What do you think about and value *outside* of your role of family mediator?" I asked after several months of listening to Adam describe the way he selflessly focused on his parents' welfare, while neglecting his own needs.

"Music and art," he replied.

"You can bring into therapy the music and art that moves you," I said.

But before Adam started doing that, there was an oral exam I had to pass: Did I empathize with his alienation from a world that "was only interested in the 'image' or 'the hype' and didn't value what was really important?"

Adam took a tack with me that had gotten him into trouble at school, religious instruction, and at home. "This culture doesn't really care about what's real and has depth, only superficial crap," he asserted. "It indoctrinates you with the idea that happiness is dependent on how much money you have and encourages people to accumulate stuff they don't need."

I could see Adam eyeing me.

"You don't find any value in self-aggrandizing artistic performers and athletes of little substance and sometimes questionable ethics?" I asked.

Adam chuckled.

"I'm envious of you," he said. "When you were my age there were more role models. We don't have that as much. You really can't find a lot of direction or inspiration from the people in the news."

Adam began bringing in journals filled with art and CDs of rock and folk music. As we explored the meaning of some of the themes in the art and music, his own unique artistic voice slowly emerged. And as he began to turn his attention to creating and expressing his vision, he was more passionate and joyful. His depression lifted and he became excited about wanting to live. He related in a more open and less constricted manner. He eventually found a girlfriend who also felt like a soul mate—a "creative outsider"—who valued his sensitivity and intelligence.

I ran into Adam on the train several years later during a semester break from college. He had learned a new foreign language and had spent the past year studying art history in Europe. He was majoring in music, fully engaged in a stimulating and creative life.

Several years later I ran into his mother. He had gotten married to his friend the creative outsider and was pursuing a career as a jazz musician.

If I treated Lawrence today, I might do several additional things. Drawing on a fundamental principle from Tibetan Buddhism—the "four reflections that turn the mind toward the Dharma"—I might ask him to meditate on his precious human birth as a gift and blessing, rather than taking it for granted and assuming it will always be there. I might also recommend that he reflect on his talents and good deeds, and on those things that he is grateful for. And I might ask him to imagine himself on his deathbed looking back on his life. What is of greatest value? Had he lived so that he had no regrets? When death comes how would he want to meet it?

References

American Foundation for Suicide Prevention. https://afsp.org/suicide-statistics/
Ueshiba, Morihei. *The Art of Peace*. Translated by John Stevens. Boston: Shambhala, 2002.

10 Our Symptoms Are Our Teachers

The Man Who Gave Birth to His Wife

Several months into therapy, on the eve of his 39th birthday, Marty, a friendly, easy-going teacher and novelist, had the following dream: "I am lying in a coffin. It's very dark, but I can see thin shafts of light through pin-prick-sized holes in the casket. No one knows that I'm there."

The dream terrified him.

"My wife says that fatal illnesses sometimes first show up in dreams."

With his neat salt-and-pepper beard, tweed jacket, button-down shirt and khaki pants, Marty looked like what he was: an Ivy-league professor. In fact, he was a tenured, highly regarded teacher of creative writing.

"Is the dream suggesting I am dying?" he asked.

"Or buried alive," I said.

"Alive, but not really living," he replied. "I write and work out, teach classes and go to the movies, but something is off, missing."

His voice trailed off and his concentration seemed to wane. There wasn't much color in his face. He looked pale and lost, almost defeated.

Marty had initiated therapy three months before because he had become very depressed for no apparent reason and was "having a hard time feeling any enthusiasm for life." He had no associations to "coffin" or "light." Shaft made him think of "being shafted" as well as "taken advantage of, taken for a ride." Taken for a ride reminded him of a dream he had several months before in which he drove around in circles in an empty parking lot. Driving around in circles made him think of a movie by Werner Herzog. "Did you ever see *Heart of Glass?*" he asked.

"No, but I've read about it," I replied. "That's the movie in which Herzog hypnotized all the actors in the movie except the sage. So, in essence all the other actors sleepwalked through the film."

"What I'm doing in my life," he said. "That makes me think of a story I never finished entitled 'The Man Who Wasn't There,' about a guy who is competent and well-liked, and seems to be all there, but is really absent from his own life."

"What's perplexing about the dream and these associations is that I just wrote an email to my best friend that my life is going well. I recently published

DOI: 10.4324/9781003604730-11

a critically acclaimed novel, and I love my wife, who is happily pursuing her passions like organic gardening and photography and recently launched a new career as a writer after a long period of struggling to find her way."

"Do I hear a *but* in your voice amid the good news?" I asked.

"Well, the dream, the story, and my associations don't exactly portray nirvana," he said.

For the next several sessions, we painstakingly reflected upon the meaning of the dream, his half-finished story, and his associations to both, linking them to their earlier sources, connecting them to his current life and his discontent, and reflecting on what they might mean to him. What slowly emerged were other, discrepant images about his life.

A highly intelligent and perceptive man, Marty was consistently drawn to a series of people who saw him as a sympathetic and caring and responded to his warmth and kindness but gave him little in return. The departmental secretary with the troubled nephew, the colleague in the throes of a mid-life crisis, the librarian whose husband was ill, a guy at the gym whose daughter was having trouble writing a college essay—all had Marty's ear, his time, and his compassion. He admitted that he felt responsible for providing sensible help or advice. He inevitably tried to heal or rescue them, which was to some extent gratifying, but left him emotionally drained and deprived.

Sadly, Marty did not recognize that often no one would ask how he was doing, or how his work was going. After one session during which he'd described a particularly exhausting day, I asked him if anyone had been there for him that day.

"My wife Caron made me a really nice breakfast," he said, after a silence.

"What happened the rest of the day?"

Marty sighed deeply. Then he stared at the wall and began speaking.

"I ran into the usual suspects." He paused with a wry smile.

"And?"

Marty thought for a couple of seconds. "I saw the reference librarian and I asked her about her husband, who had surgery two weeks ago. She told me he was doing really well, and then she said, 'Nice talking with you,' and she walked away, and I walked into my classroom."

"Did she ask how you were?"

"No, but she may have had a lot to do."

"Who else are you going to 'excuse' today?" I wondered.

"After class, I saw the departmental secretary. I asked about her nephew, who she's trying to get into a drug rehabilitation program. I volunteered to call the director, who I vaguely know."

"Did she ask how you were?"

"Well, no, I could tell she wasn't feeling that great and she might be a little intimidated by me."

"Intimidated by *you*?" I asked.

"Well yes. She often makes comments about the books she sees me carrying, like she's intimidated," he said.

"Admiration or intimidation?" I asked.

"All right fine," he said. "Maybe I assume I'm making her feel bad, that it's my fault, *and* my responsibility to 'fix' it."

Marty is silent, and very still. When he speaks, his voice is low and a little hoarse.

"I don't get very much back, do I?"

The question is rhetorical, and I don't answer.

"I feel like an ass. I'm always being a nice guy, but no one cares about me. That's it, isn't it—but how do I stop being a nice guy? How do I get people to give back, ask about me?"

In addition to his constant caretaking, Marty faithfully volunteered for teaching and administrative projects that didn't really stimulate or challenge him. These commitments filled up his time. This not only added to his deprivation, but it also allowed him to continually put off focusing on what he wanted and needed.

"I have a variety of interesting writing projects that I never quite finish, that remain virtual ideas, and I never seem to get to them. They're buried away in my study, under piles of this other stuff I can't seem to get out of doing," he said.

Like him in the coffin, I thought.

Marty was a caretaker *par excellence*, who accommodated to the needs of others—almost compulsively giving them what they wanted—which often left him feeling neglected and deprived in his life and career.

When Marty wasn't taking care of other people—solving their problems and ministering to their needs—he was writing. But as he recounted his professional "achievements" to me—he was the author of two well-received novels and was well-liked as a teacher—he seemed to be describing someone else. I wasn't surprised that he derived little satisfaction from his successes—he spoke as if he didn't have them. And then there was the small matter that despite his achievements, he also "had not really found his voice or tapped into his potential."

How could he? I thought. *He has structured his life so that there is no time for what really matters to him.*

In a session several months into therapy, Marty discussed the "gap" between what other people thought of him and how he saw himself.

"There's another story I never completed, 'The Double,' about a man who doesn't appreciate his own value and takes himself for granted," he said.

"Isn't there a novella by Dostoevsky entitled *The Double* (1846/2009), *about a man whose double shows up at work and persecuted him?" I asked.*

"Yes," Marty says. "But mine is different. The main character is not split in two like Golyadkin in Dostoevsky's story, and only realizes, as he is dying, that while the world has seen him as a Goliath he has always felt like a Lilliputian—a shadow of himself, a man who is not fully inhabiting his life."

As my understanding of Marty's childhood deepened, the links between the story and his life became clearer. Marty was the youngest of two siblings who grew up in a small northeastern town. He was three years younger than his sister Betsy, who was a "pistol." She was bright, nervous, edgy, self-involved, and perpetually dissatisfied, and had severe emotional problems, the origin of which Marty couldn't pin-point. From what we could reconstruct, she was an abrasive person who had adversarial relationships with friends and family alike. From Marty's perspective she was like an "independent operative" within their family. She did what she wanted and was responsible to no one. Betsy treated other people like they were simply objects in her quest to fulfill her own needs.

Marty's parents didn't know what to do with Betsy. Nothing they tried—from understanding to tough love—had any positive impact. Marty's efforts were also to no avail. But that didn't stop him from feeling guilt and a profound sense of failure for not being able to get through to her.

In high school Betsy began abusing pot, alcohol, and a host of other substances. She withdrew more and more from Marty and her parents. After high school she went to college in Southern California and the schism between her and her family widened. At first Marty tried to keep in touch, but Betsy didn't reciprocate. As adults they have had little contact. Marty eventually became tired of trying to bail Betsy out of one jam after another.

As Marty recounted how bad he felt for not having any lasting impact on Betsy's downward trajectory, I knew we'd have to explore whether compulsively helping people in need was a way of doing penance for the imagined "crime" of not rescuing his troubled sister.

Marty's relationship with his parents was also problematic.

At the beginning of treatment, he described his mother as caring and devoted and his father as critical and remote. As treatment proceeded, other images emerged. He eventually realized his mother was a rigid person who demanded that everyone around her live in accordance with her narrow view of reality which was ruled by "fortune cookie" axioms. Clichéd responses ("You must have felt bad when you got that rejection") replaced genuine emotional engagement. Talking to his mother resembled verbal fencing; "she parries everything I say." Instead of being affirmed and validated by her, Marty felt literally invisible in her presence, almost as if she looked through him, not at him.

Marty had a distant relationship with his father, a small business owner who was intelligent and detached, critical and passive. His father submitted to his wife's way of living and relating, and never sustained an interest in Marty's life. "They were like an impenetrable united front," he said. While he knew that his father loved him, Marty had no memories of ever feeling protected or supported by him.

In Marty's view, he had to "harmonize" with his parent's view of reality. That was his only hope of being emotionally related to them.

His parents didn't talk with him about his world, his plans, his hopes, or his fears. When he tried to tell them about something good in his life, his mother would listen briefly and then change the subject and begin talking about a small achievement of a child of a friend. Marty's father asked him the same questions over and over about his life as if Marty didn't exist in his father's consciousness and the latter was making "small talk with a stranger."

Marty got the distinct impression that his parents seemed happiest when he was dependent on them. To keep the peace, his life had to revolve around their needs. As a result, his needs got little attention, and he learned few life skills that would allow him to develop an independent existence.

Marty survived by latching on to two older males—a history teacher and a baseball coach—who appreciated and supported his burgeoning academic and athletic talents. Books became his salvation; a way of trying to fill in the missing gaps in his life and figuring out how to live. Academic success became his ticket out; winning a scholarship to a good university was a way of being more independent and escaping the deadening atmosphere in his family.

Marty developed a private world of depth and richness, but because his parents never "saw" or appreciated who he was, he was never able to accurately see himself. A superior student and a gifted writer, who didn't realize the value of his "voice," Marty was excessively modest, never appreciating or talking about his academic interests or accomplishments. It was not surprising that he underestimated his potential. Marty became an overachiever who was convinced that he was a failure. He also had great difficulty believing in the validity of his perceptions and beliefs and sustaining a commitment to them.

The major means Marty used to gain an identity was by giving to other people. Being a gifted caretaker of the emotionally needy replaced what would normally have been the pursuit of his own dreams. But in his accommodation to other people he neglected his own needs and interests. This left him feeling directionless, which led to a sense that "something was missing" in his life.

When he began dating in high school, a disturbing pattern developed. He mostly went out with "wounded sparrows"—girls with "handicaps." One was a lost soul from a severely dysfunctional family with an insatiable need for being appreciated and catered to; another was a rebellious and alienated outcast who tried to monopolize all his time and attention and undermine his relationships with male friends. The glue that held these relationships together was the energy Marty devoted to trying to heal them, which left him deprived and neglected.

Marty described a positive relationship with his wife, Caron, a loving and supportive partner who really understood and appreciated him. Given Marty's family history—and his tendency to take care of "wounded sparrows," I wasn't surprised to learn that Caron was a deeply traumatized and self-neglectful person when he first met her 20 years ago. Caron was a highly gifted musician as a child, who apparently did not fulfill the promise of her talent because of parental neglect.

Caron's father was extremely bright but very damaged. A deeply neglected and suspicious man, he became a ruthless narcissist who eventually abandoned his family when Caron was a junior in high school. Caron's family lived on the edge of poverty while her father was living well in the same town.

Caron's mother was an intelligent and depressed person who had her hands full raising her three children. She emotionally neglected Caron, her oldest daughter.

Her parents offered no support, interest, or guidance regarding her musical interests—especially singing. Because of the absence of backing, she didn't take her passions and talents seriously.

Caron learned to give compulsively to others and disregard—and expect little for—herself. She became a highly skilled nurturer, who gave to others as a way of feeling valued.

Most people saw Caron as a kind, nurturing, and selfless person who didn't care for herself. But underneath her selfless persona Marty saw a feisty soul with great intellectual and artistic potential. From the beginning of their marriage, he had committed himself to helping Caron trust her perceptions and value herself, pursue her passions and bring out her voice. From what I could gather, he did this in several ways. He spent a great deal of time listening to her unique view of people and the world. No one had ever taken the time to take her seriously. In her previous relationships she had played second-fiddle to dominating men. Marty also encouraged Caron to pursue her passions like photography and gardening. Caron's tendency was to sprint out of the starting gate; she would take up a hobby with great enthusiasm only to lose interest or not follow through. Not only was Marty often there to cheer her on, but he also taught her how to be disciplined and focused and to take her interests more seriously. To support her he sometimes joined her activities—even when he wasn't particularly interested in them.

On Marty's 40th birthday, Caron wrote in a card to him:

You've given me:
 love,
 support
 understanding,
 high ceilings and fresh breezes,
 a few sleepless nights,
 a wonderful deepening understanding of things I never knew existed,
 my voice
 love,
 c

Marty's devotion to his wife eventually paid off. Caron started taking her emotions and needs more seriously. As she began pursuing old and long-buried passions and gave voice to herself, her native artistic and intellectual talents emerged. One day Marty came home earlier from work than he had planned, and Caron was serenading the shower. It was the first time he had heard her beautiful and richly timbered voice in 20 years.

A few years earlier, an old friend of Marty's, a scholar of Greek and Roman mythology, who knew Caron when Marty first met her, said to him, "When I first met Caron, she was quiet and reserved. She's completely different now. You've helped her find her voice."

But the terrible irony was that Marty, who gave birth to his wife, was not fully born himself.

On the eve of his 40th birthday Marty indicated that he felt a good deal better than he did a year ago when he first came to therapy. But while his depression and malaise had lifted, he was troubled because he had difficulty completing a project that meant a lot to him. Working with a dream clarified where Marty was stuck in his life: "I met with a book publisher who was interested in a collection of short stories I've been working on, entitled 'How the Nightingale Found Her Voice.' He is pressuring me for the finished manuscript which is long overdue. But I don't have it. And I believed I never would. I am stuck and confused. The publisher is quite disappointed."

Marty drew a blank when we explored being "stuck and confused." His association to the undelivered book, however, opened up new pathways.

"I have completed most of the book except the title story. I just don't understand why I can't finish it. I think I know the story and where it is going—it's about a woman with a beautiful voice who was not able to sing for many years, until, through the love of her husband, she came into her own and found her 'voice.' It's in part a fictionalized account of me and Caron," Marty said.

However, the obstacle to completing the story remained a mystery until Marty described the underlying theme of "How the Nightingale Found Her Voice" in greater detail. "It's about the 'fruits' of transformation—what it means to sing, to flourish, to bring out one's voice," he said.

Is he having so much trouble completing the story because he is trying to write about his own unfinished transformation? "Maybe the story isn't only or really about Caron," I said.

"What do you mean—who could it be about?" he asked.

I am silent.

"Me?" he asked incredulously.

"Maybe you're stuck about what it means to 'sing' and can't finish it because you haven't experienced it—you have to complete certain changes in your life so that *you* are freed up to bring out your voice," I said.

The professor was very still. And pensive. After a long silence he said, "I was a midwife to my wife's birth, but I'm still buried alive myself. The story I haven't written is *my* life! The man who gave birth to his wife needs to come alive himself!"

In Marty's case, this process of awakening and integration took place over time and happened in two stages. First, he had to transform the familiar, ingrained patterns of "neglecting himself" and "healing wounded sparrows." Then he had to create something new—build a life in which his passion, vision, and goals played a more central role.

Marty was one of those few who treated other people better than they treated themselves. "The old me was a non-existent me," he said. "There for others, neglecting myself."

"You are nicer to other people than you are to yourself," I said to him on more than one occasion.

As Marty felt increasingly understood by me, he began trusting his own perceptions and valuing himself. When he finally realized how overinvested he was in other people's problems—and that this entailed neglecting his own—he made powerful inroads in taking himself more seriously. Over time he learned to challenge his tendency to devalue himself and participate in one-way, depriving relationships.

He began asking himself questions:

"Am I getting together with this person because I value the friendship and I'm getting something significant back or because I am guilty and don't want to hurt their feelings?"

"Am I taking on a project because it would be stimulating—or because I can't say no and don't want to let anyone down?"

These helped him avoid situations in which he would compulsively take care of other people and leave himself out.

"I used to see life as a choice between two deadly options," Marty said, "Being connected to other people, but losing myself, or being myself but being alone. In my work with you I've learned there's a third option: being myself while being connected with other people, but the 'right people'—the friends who really care about me the way I care about them."

Over the next few months, he renewed contact with and deepened two old friendships that had been a source of support and stimulation that he had drifted from over the years. These friends shared and affirmed what really mattered to him—the search for wisdom and health of mind and body, friendship and making the world a more humane place.

Changing his life was not always a smooth process for Marty. During one session, he described feeling uncertainty and fear. "I know my life is improving, but in some way I am more lost. There's a vacuum."

"There's often a void, even a 'death,' when we change, let go of long-standing patterns," I said. "A death to who we thought we were and how we relate to ourselves and to other people."

"Funny you should say that," he replied. "I've been having images and fantasies of disaster and death recently. Not death, exactly . . . no . . . more like landscapes of doom and barrenness. Really being authentically myself—fully being who I am—is like entering a post-apocalyptic universe of desolation, aloneness, and sterility."

"How do you fill the void—where's the blueprint for who I really am?" Marty asked. "Where, in the past, do we find this counsel?"

"It's tempting to search for an earlier, more authentic version of the 'real you'—a True Self in your past—that provides guidance and direction," I said. "Such a version of yourself is presumed to provide a specific map for how you should live. But there is no True Self waiting to be found underneath your long-standing tendency toward inauthenticity and compliance. Behind this false outer shell is an undeveloped, inchoate sense of self. Therapy involves building on and developing this self."

From then on Marty and I focused on *self-creation* in the present—constructing a new life through ongoing self-examination, and new kinds of relationships and commitments based on his authentic values, goals, and interests.

There is much emphasis in our age on "just doing it"—for example, simply being yourself. For Marty, like for many of us, it was not so easy.

The biggest obstacle was his continuing tendency to accommodate to the needs of other people and neglect himself. We were able to resolve this long-standing pattern by exploring the way he played it out with me. It felt very good to be with Marty—so good that I began to get curious about it. I noticed that he always gave me the benefit of the doubt—even when I didn't necessarily deserve it—and he never seemed to disagree with or be upset with me. I realized that my feeling of success and ease in our relationship signaled, not that the therapy was always proceeding in a completely positive manner, but that he was habitually conforming to what he assumed I wanted. My comfort with him was as much a result of Marty's accommodating to me, as it was an indication of the success of the therapy. Attention to this pattern between us aided Marty in eventually understanding and shedding his compliance.

As Marty was increasingly authentic with me, it made it much easier to be genuine with other people. Conserving his resources more wisely—engaging in fewer rescue missions for Betsy-surrogates, living authentically, and reconnecting with nurturing friends—all freed Marty up to pursue his own passions and interests. This was a crucial part of creating himself— and his life—anew.

As his trust in himself expanded even further, Marty resumed several old passions—especially long-distance running and yoga. He slowly began to really savor his abilities and give himself sufficient time to exercise them. Over the following months he got deeper into writing, finishing two manuscripts that had been half-completed for several years, including *How the Nightingale Found Her Voice*.

The man who gave birth to his wife was now more fully alive himself.

Reference

Dostoevsky, Fyodor. *The Double*. Translated by Richard Pevear and Larissa Volokhonsky. New York: Knopf, 2009. (Original work published 1846)

11 On Being a Zen Psychoanalyst
The Union of Presence, Meaning, and Intimacy

"You know, you're a Zen guy," a patient who was a Roshi—a Zen master—said to me after the first several weeks of treatment many years ago.

"What *is* Zen?" a snarky middle-aged man asked me around the same time, as I walked past him leaving the gym.

"It began many centuries ago in China . . ." I said, in a remarkably un-Zen-like response.

"Gimme the short version," he shot back.

"Did you have coffee this morning?" I asked.

"Yeah." He raised his Styrofoam cup.

"Did you really taste it, or were you a million miles away?"

"I really tasted it."

"That's Zen," I said.

"Okay, I can go with that."

"Zen is teaching adults what comes naturally to children," I added as I left the gym.

The process of "growing up" into an adult—learning a language and becoming adept at categorizing the world and mastering the rules and roles that make up the culture we are part of—alienates us from ourselves and a natural, spontaneous, and authentic way of being. We lose our childhood innocence in our quest to earn a living and succeed at work, find a mate and raise a family.

Zen meditation opens up our latent capacity for freshness of perception, wonder, and delight. Not only do we become more open and receptive to the world, but we are also capable of bearing witness to a greater range of human experience. This is, in and of itself, wonderfully "therapeutic."

A student of Zen met with a venerable Zen teacher and told him he was riddled with depression and fear. The Roshi, or honored teacher, recommended "Zen therapy." "When you completely listen to the sound of the birds where is your depression?" the Zen master asked. "When you chop vegetables where is your fear?"

To a Western-trained psychotherapist this is intriguing, if unusual, advice. Much of the time therapists, as well as the people they work with, sleepwalk

DOI: 10.4324/9781003604730-12

through their days—lost in ruminative thoughts, pointless worries, and countless pseudo-problems. Meanwhile, we suffer unnecessarily and miss so much. The lives of psychotherapists, as well as clients in therapy, would be greatly enhanced if they spent more time directly engaging in their experiences. Fears about the future and regrets from the past would both lessen if we followed the Roshi's advice.

The Roshi's "Zen therapy" left me with several questions: Is merging with whatever we encounter enough? Is it ever too narrow? Is there a shadow side to it?

Most people cannot continuously be one with their experience. Even the meditatively trained spend an inordinate amount of time in their heads, disconnected from life, worrying about what hasn't happened and regretting what has. So, depression and fear, guilt and shame will return.

And emotions, as I (Rubin, 2011) suggested in *The Art of Flourishing*, are feedback about what we value and struggle with. Even if we could merge without interruption with the song of the birds or cutting veggies, it would interfere with learning what our emotions are communicating. Anger can signal hurt; jealousy tells us what we want more of in our lives. Healing our wounds and conflicts lies in integrating our feelings, which entails understanding them, not simply merging with them.

In his own life, the Roshi's "medicine" of Zen therapy didn't quite suffice: He was embroiled in sexual abuse scandals—"molesting or coercing hundreds of others into having sexual contact with him during one-on-one training sessions at his Rinzai-ji Zen Center in Los Angeles and at his retreat camps," as Paul Vitello reported in the *New York Times* on August 4, 2014. "An independent panel of Buddhist leaders concluded in 2013. . . that students had complained to Mr. Sasaki's staff about his behavior since the early 1970s, and that those 'who chose to speak out were silenced, exiled, ridiculed or otherwise punished,'" Vitello (2014) added.

One way of salvaging the valuable aspects of the Zen master's insights about "Zen therapy" is to integrate them with two hallmarks of psychoanalysis, namely the search for meaning and the focus on *relationality*; the importance in human development and the therapeutic process of our relationships, real and fantasied, external and internalized. Psychoanalysts devote a great deal of attention to illuminating the meaning of whatever symptoms and symbols patients bring to treatment. While Zen can be highly therapeutic, what the Roshi recommended as "Zen therapy" is not truly *therapy* unless it focuses on meaning, as well as merging with and becoming deeply connected to what we encounter. Buddhism neglects meaning.

One of Freud's towering insights (1900) was that people grow ill—and suffer from—experiences that they don't understand. "Find out about the parent they don't talk about, not the one they do," a Freudian supervisor of mine once aptly noted. While humans have an infinite capacity for self-deception, we also have a remarkable ability to communicate what troubles and haunts us in symbols, dreams, and symptoms. These offer clues: breadcrumbs leading those who listen attentively to the source and current manifestation of our problems in living.

To understand these clues, we have to illuminate their symbolic meaning, which occurs on various levels at once. That is one of the great therapeutic discoveries.

Bringing Zen and Psychoanalysis Together

Returning to the title of this chapter, I didn't think of myself as a Zen psychoanalyst until my patient, the Zen master, said to me: "You're a Zen guy."

Being a "Zen psychoanalyst," just like working with a Zen koan, has two aspects: realization and actualization. We need to understand, explain, and then practice and embody it. I will first present the spirit of how I work—briefly describing aspects of three cases—and then I will attempt to shed light from the other side of the couch.

All Psychiatrists are Assholes

They sat on my couch: the prospective patient, a brilliant and cantankerous 13-year-old boy/man; and his mother, a lawyer. Actually, she sat, and he fidgeted and sank down, at one point putting his head on her lap. She was at her wit's end: her husband had killed himself the year before, and her son, a precocious and utterly demoralized adolescent, was desolate and depressed to the point of being suicidal.

She did most of the talking, filling in the horrific details of the tragedy she and her son had endured in the past year. They had both lost the person most important to them, a larger-than-life man with a commanding personality and titanic intellect, who alternately stimulated, challenged, and fiercely loved his son. The boy said very little. He was busy checking me out, gauging whether I could be trusted. He had spent the previous year seeing a variety of psychiatrists and psychologists, none of whom he had connected with.

As I ended the session, I caught a fleeting glimpse of the statue of the Buddha on the windowsill of my office, his face eclipsed by a curtain obscuring his beatific smile. I got up from my chair and stood near the door. My prospective patient lumbered toward me, his mother at his flank.

"All psychiatrists are assholes," he informed me.

"There are two problems with your statement," I said. "One, I am a psychoanalyst, not a psychiatrist. Two, given your supposed intelligence—why did it take you so long to figure out my limitations?"

"I'm going to poison my mother," my psychiatry-loving patient said, upping the ante.

"Thank you," I said.

"You can't say thank you, you're a shrink," he replied, momentarily flustered, trying for damage control.

"Well, *you've* given *me* a new strategy I can employ against stubborn teenage boys," I told him.

The tiny half-smile on the right side of his mouth conceded round two.

I didn't consciously plan my response. If I had, my guess is that it probably would have been canned and mannered, off base and not very helpful. When Max challenged me at the door my mind was empty, free of preconceptions, receptive to his tone of voice and the humor—and vulnerability—underneath his apparent hostility. It can be scary to be without a map or a compass, to not have a particular theory or set response to draw on. I didn't mind. My experience over the years has cultivated a deep faith in the capacity of patients to creatively communicate what they feel and need, drawing a picture with their actions and words of what they cannot always verbally say. My capacity to hear and see what they were trying to tell me has infinitely increased when I put aside both what I thought I knew and any preconceived ideas about how therapy should proceed. And that provided access to a remarkably ingenious state of mind I mentioned in Chapter 2, *mushin*, or *no-mindedness*—what D.T. Suzuki (1971) in *Zen and Japanese Culture* described as awareness-without-self-consciousness, which leads to greater freedom and creativity.

Torn Checks and Chinese Doctors

They are on the edge of divorce. Ellen, a small woman with a loud voice, was fed up with Gus, her husband, a burly man who said very little. With barely concealed hostility she told me that he refused to talk about what's bothering him, drank too much, and worked long hours at a job with poor compensation. Ellen wanted Gus to leave their home, but he refused.

They had been married for several years and had two young children. Each worked. While there was evidently some affection between them, the problems that brought them into therapy had been there from the beginning of the relationship.

Their issues mirrored the difficulties their parents had. Ellen's mother and father had gotten divorced when she was young. Her father drank too much, cared about his family but was overly judgmental of Ellen and her mother and emotionally distant. Gus's parents were still together, but his father was a highly critical man who beat down his son, drank too much, and was withdrawn from his wife. Gus's besieged mother passively endured her husband's behavior and failed to protect or support her son. Gus grew up feeling devalued and deprived. He had to bury his anger; to express it would incur his father's wrath.

In the first several sessions we danced around on the surface. I slowly got the lay of the land—the fear and misgivings and self-protectiveness. Building trust with each of them took time and patience. Once they both felt safer, I made tentative forays into deeper and rougher waters. Eventually we hit pay dirt—the essential issues that were troubling them. But this was no panacea.

Actually, they felt worse—rawer and more vulnerable. I had questions. Would I be able to help them? Would they stay stuck in the misery that brought them to me? Would they each be able to make the necessary changes? Would they discover that their original dreams of escaping the prison and pain of their families of origin were merely mirages, pipe dreams?

Like many couples, at this point they pulled back, dug in, reverted to old, dysfunctional coping strategies, protecting themselves against the break-throughs they hungered for and were terrified by.

In the next few sessions, we expanded our exploration of the themes that surfaced in the first session. Ellen was intensely deprived and harbored a lot of resentment, which she wasn't shy about expressing. Gus said that she was angry and hostile—"ranting and raving." That caused him to shut down, dive into work—the one area of life that offered any satisfaction—and anaesthe-tize his pain through alcohol. This only exacerbated her dissatisfaction and attacks. But underneath Ellen's anger with Gus for working at a dead-end job, his drinking, and his absence from home, was love for him and a wish that someone could get through his nearly impenetrable wall.

The next session was a nightmare. Gus had no interest in psychotherapy. He silently glared at Ellen, who desperately wanted to go around the wall he continually erected. I sensed that she longed to be closer to her angry and withdrawn husband. Softness and kindness, exasperation, and impatience, she had tried it all. None of these things had made a dent in Mr. Locked Vault.

The session had resembled a crowded urban center at rush hour—heavy doses of congestion, gridlock, and simmering rage. Gus had spent our entire time together quietly sabotaging any efforts to break through the distance between him and his wife. He had successfully stymied both her and my best efforts at improving their rocky relationship. I was very frustrated.

He stood abruptly at the end of the session and handed me a check. *For what?* I remembered thinking. *Nothing constructive happened in the session.* I don't know what possessed me, but I tore the check in half and threw the pieces in the air. They fluttered down and landed on the floor between us. Gus stared at me, ready to escalate. I didn't blame him. I wondered if I had finally gone too far.

"I've been told that in ancient China, a doctor only got paid when he helped his patient," I said. "We got nowhere during this session because you interfered with my doing my job. So, I can't in good conscience accept your check. It would be immoral."

Gus glared at me, turned, and left without a word.

I can't remember if he ever replaced the check, but the next week he came back with Ellen, which surprised me, and dove into the session, which shocked me. He took an active role, sharing his emotions—including what Ellen did that hurt him—and struggled to understand his life and marriage. He was less hostile and more related.

Their unspoken pact was also revealed. While they seemed to want to improve the relationship, they also didn't really believe it was possible.

So, they had settled for a co-existence that protected them against being vulnerable or rejected, but that avoided deeper intimacy. In fact, they had given up on the possibility of a closer relationship, settling for whatever emotional scraps they could get.

In the following sessions they each began seeing patterns from the past that interfered with being closer. Ellen realized that she was criticizing Gus the way her father had picked her apart and her mother had put down her father. Gus acknowledged that he was passively resisting Ellen the way his father had opposed his mother. Gus and Ellen also became more sensitive to dysfunctional patterns in the present. Ellen recognized how her criticalness and impatience contributed to Gus being angry and withdrawn. Gus realized how his passivity made Ellen believe that she didn't have a partner.

Over time their relationship improved. Conflict didn't disappear, but they handled it much more constructively, listening to and respecting each other. Ellen practiced treating Gus more patiently and kindly. Gus worked on his drinking and learned to express his hurt and anger more directly and to respond to her efforts to connect. She learned how difficult it was for him to do this and that it was not always her fault that he could not. They each forgave mistakes, dropped grudges, and even compromised. And when that didn't work, a dose of humor helped them ride the waves of the difficult times. They started having more fun together, appreciating their differences.

I am not normally in the business of tearing up checks. But when I tried to explore Gus's rage and obstructionist behavior verbally, he denied it and battled with me and we, like he and Ellen, were stymied.

There is no single way to get through to a difficult or hostile person. Empathy sometimes makes them feel understood and validated, melting their anger and antagonism. At other times, they may want to hold onto rather than resolve or give up their anger. Conflict can be a way of protesting against or sabotaging those people one is disappointed with. It can also protect against intimacy when one is frightened of closeness. For many people, hostility makes them feel stronger and less vulnerable than feeling hurt.

When a person is attached to anger, you may get nowhere with empathy or understanding. If they are invested in punishing you, you are not playing on a level playing field. Resolving sticky issues is often not a high priority for them.

They can't always be approached rationally or logically. When you do, you get thwarted.

Sometimes mental jujitsu, a kind of turning things upside down so the difficult person gets a completely different picture of what they are doing, may be necessary. This often wakes them up and points toward a way out of the state they are stuck in. Words were worthless currency to Gus—he was skilled at parrying or ignoring them. Tearing up the check seemed a more powerful and effective way of holding up a mirror to his anger and oppositional behavior than *talking* about it. The torn check was a dramatic way of showing him that he was not getting what he was paying for—and that *he* was responsible for changing it.

It is generally accepted among psychotherapists of different theoretical orientations that *action* is an important medium through which clients communicate with their therapist. Clients not only anticipate that the therapist will react to them and treat them like significant people in their past did, but they also often unwittingly *do* things to elicit similar responses. For example, Gus not only assumed that Ellen would criticize him, but he also provoked her into acting like the nag he detested.

It's a timeworn therapeutic truism that the therapist's verbal interpretations or explanations—linking the client's behavior in the present to hidden thoughts, emotions, or fantasies in the past—fuels change. What has been less recognized is that a therapist's *actions* in therapy are often a powerful means for communication and transformation. What the torn check illustrates is that *interventions*—what the therapist does—can sometimes be as effective as what they say. Interventions—conveyed through facial expressions and tone of voice, humor and laughter—may communicate to the client what might not be expressible by words alone. And they often break through an emotional logjam and bypass a person's resistance, as they did with Gus.

Tearing up Gus's check or meeting Max's attack on psychiatrists with irreverent humor were interventions that communicated something vital about my understanding of each person and our relationship. These interventions removed potential roadblocks to greater intimacy between us and opened up new possibilities for healing.

Sixteen years later Ellen called me. Their son was thriving and applying to college. Gus had been "clean and sober" for 16 years and liked his new work, which offered a retirement and health plan. Ellen was fulfilled in her work and her life, and she and Gus really enjoyed each other. They hardly ever fought, and when they did they quickly resolved it.

"Everyone said we'd never make it," she told me. "If not for you we wouldn't have."

I am silent and deeply touched, I notice a rush of energy course through me as she is saying this; never having realized the impact our work had on them.

"When we first came for therapy, I wanted a divorce and I wanted you to tell him to leave," Ellen said. "I'm glad you didn't. And I'm glad Gus stuck with me. Now we are the happiest and most in love we have ever been."

Discovering Meaning

For me, the heart of being a Zen psychoanalyst is merging with what life presents—like the Roshi recommended—figuring out what the client's words and behaviors mean and responding un-self-consciously and wholeheartedly.

It is infinitely harder to merge with a painful emotion than with the song of the birds, although the process is the same. What I call *training meditation-in-action* offers a means of practicing this in stages. First, we can open to sights and sounds that are either pleasing or neutral by attempting to be one with them and savor them and soak them in. This develops concentration and equanimity, which can serve as a foundation to merge with pleasant or neutral physical sensations. Once that is manageable—whether it takes minutes or days, weeks or months—the meditator/therapist can practice becoming one with more challenging physical sensations. Eventually we can merge with physical pain. We can then practice merging with pleasant or less afflictive emotions (such as disappointment and minor anxiety). Then we can tackle slightly more challenging feelings. Eventually we can practice merging with anger, guilt, and fear—and later shame.

Discovering meaning is the second aspect of Zen psychoanalysis. Meaning can be confusing because it is sometimes disguised and often can't be read on the surface. Decoding is often necessary.

We never know the meaning of something in advance. "What is the meaning of such [flying] dreams?" asked Freud in *The Interpretation of Dreams* (1900). "It is impossible to give a general reply. As we shall hear, they mean something different in every instance . . ."

Meaning is arrived at, as Freud (1900) recognized, not by translating what you are examining into what you already know or assume, no matter what school of psychoanalysis or psychotherapy inspires you, but by eliciting the person's unique associations or reactions to it. Otherwise, you interpret "into" the experience what cannot be interpreted "from" it.

We find meaning by paying attention to and being one with the *cause* and the *function* (or purpose) of a thought, feeling, or action, which includes the newly emergent potentials it embodies. Listening deeply on two levels or channels at once—conscious and unconscious—is indispensable. Meditation neglects the latter, as I wrote (Rubin, 2009) in "Deepening Psychoanalytic Listening: The Marriage of Buddha and Freud."

Sometimes meaning emerges directly and automatically when we are truly one with what we are encountering—like my playful encounter with the bereft teenager or tearing up Gus's check in the face of his obstructive behavior. Zen calls this *prajna* wisdom or intuition. A direct perception leads to an unself-conscious and whole-hearted response. Then the analyst is a *jazz improviser*, who has mastered the fundamentals of the therapeutic process and is flexible and adaptable in the present (Rubin, 1998). This is the third aspect of Zen psychoanalysis, which we'll explore shortly.

Sometimes oneness is not enough to determine meaning and one needs to step back from direct contact with a person or emotion and reflect on it—what I call *reflective intimacy* in my book *Practicing Meditative Psychotherapy* (Rubin, 2013).

What did my teenage patient mean when he said, "All psychiatrists are assholes" and why did he say it? On the surface his remark might seem angry and hostile, a direct attack. He had just met me, yet he was making a blanket and provocative statement that I was a jerk. I heard what he said, not as an affront, but as an expression of his feeling that he's not enamored of therapists. But why? Was this his experience? I thought he was asking several questions: How free and safe is it in the session for him to be himself? Could I deal with his rage and impotent confusion? Am I an authoritarian who will retaliate if he's real or hostile?

But there was even more to it. Was he pushing me away because he was afraid of getting close, relying on me, and then being abandoned like his father left him? Or had he become like his father, a highly critical person who was never satisfied with anything? Was he treating me the way he had been treated? Or was he feeling safe enough to say that psychiatrists, as well as mothers and fathers, had profoundly let him down?

As I listened to my young patient, I heard a soul in trouble, a person who had been devastated, and perhaps more importantly had not been encouraged to mourn his loss. He was literally imploding under the house arrest inadvertently imposed by his bereft mother, who was facing her own personal nightmare and didn't have the energy to handle his rage and torment. He felt "poisoned" by both his father's death and his mother's failure to help him face it. He longed for an opportunity to have his pain witnessed and validated. So, when he challenged me, I heard it as an expression of how he felt and a "test"—was it safe enough to be real? I sensed he needed me to meet his onslaught without flinching. I could have asked him if he was angry or betrayed or afraid when he said, "All psychiatrists are assholes" and "I am going to poison my mother," but I believed he needed *actions* rather than words to know it was safe to trust me and be himself.

We talked some years ago about that first session. "My statement about psychiatrists was my way of letting you know that I wouldn't defer to you because of age or stature," he said. "My statement about my mother conveyed that therapy won't fix anything, you don't have control, and I'm angry."

In retrospect, I'm glad I said "Thank you" when he said he was going to poison his mother. I was relieved that he hadn't yet given up all hope of being found on the desert island of private agony that he inhabited and very happy that he felt safe enough to challenge me and be aggressive and authentic. Meeting his challenge head-on seemed crucial to launching the therapy. Exploring his wish to poison his mother ("Why do you think you said that?" or being subtly shocked or disturbed by it) would have conveyed, I suspect, that I couldn't handle his emotions. It would have doomed the therapy from the start. My humor communicated to him that I had the endurance to handle him *and* that I liked him.

I learned recently that Max, a C+ student in high school, graduated from one of the best law schools in the world and was practicing law at a highly esteemed firm. He was following his passion, drawing on his unique strengths, and embodying his talents and skills.

Zen and Relationships

My treatment with a therapist-in-training with a severe trauma history elucidates the third aspect of being a Zen psychoanalyst—the importance of a self-reflective, empathic, and creative human relationship. Psychoanalysis enriches Zen with its provision of a collaborative bond designed to validate the client's experience and provide opportunities for new forms of relatedness and self-transformation.

During our work, after a deep connection was established and a great deal of trauma had emerged, my analysand indicated that she felt worse—and stuck. At first, we joined and directly encountered both the physical and emotional experience of each. Frozen physical energy, terror, and mental lethargy became constant companions. As we stepped back and explored her emotions, various meanings emerged—especially the way she felt in danger of being abandoned—and re-traumatized—by me. She seemed relieved, but still somewhat stymied. I eventually wondered if the closeness of our relationship was making her feel *worse* because if someone she liked and respected valued her then maybe she wasn't loathsome, which made her feel even more betrayed by her parents who didn't protect her from the abuse she was subjected to at a religious organization they sent her to.

As I continued to reflect on her predicament "Kyogen's Man Up a Tree" koan (13th century/Yamada, 1979), one of those paradoxical Zen puzzles Zen teachers give their students, came to mind. This was a question I had encountered in my own training to be a Zen teacher. A man who is in a tree, hanging from a branch by his mouth, is asked by a man under the tree, "What is the meaning of Bodhidharma's coming from the West?" (Bodhidharma is traditionally viewed as the transmitter of Buddhism from India to China). The man hanging by his mouth is in a desperate predicament. He will fail if he doesn't say something, and he will fall if he does.

We often find ourselves in a related dilemma in therapy and in our lives when we must respond to something when we seemingly can't, no good options seem available, and we don't know what to do.

Self-reflection, self-awareness, and empathy are our emotional and moral compass. What is the person struggling with? What do they need to heal or thrive? How are we impacting and fostering or interfering with the process? Knowledge of all of this aids the therapist in being more adept and creative.

My client, the therapist, like all of us, can't cure herself alone. She needed me to witness and validate her trauma and pain, yet trusting—and relying on—other people was terrifying, and her abusers threatened to kill her if she revealed what happened. I knew that she was an imaginative therapist and a talented artist who regularly drew on art—and Jung's technique of active imagination, or artistically exploring symbolic imagery in dreams—to explore her emotions. Knowing that speaking about how she was traumatized was itself traumatic, I suggested a "life koan" for her: "How can you communicate what you need to with me *without* talking about it?"

"I'll bring in artwork Friday," she said with a noticeable sigh of relief.

Friday, she brought in a brightly colored mask with a closed mouth. She took out a pen, punctured the sealed mouth and began speaking about both the way she was traumatized at a religious cult her parents sent her to, and forbidden to speak about it, as well as new aspects of her trauma and her self-silencing.

Since that time, she has spoken more freely and deeply about her traumas. She slowly healed. She has also found her voice in her psychoanalytic classes, was noticeably more engaged in treatment, and eventually completed her training and began her own practice including working with traumatized survivors of a school shooting.

These vignettes hopefully illustrate the three main elements of being a Zen psychoanalyst—the union of intimacy, meaning, and relationality. Whole-hearted and un-self-conscious connection to a bereft young man and an oppositional adult led to an emotionally intimate and unpredictable encounter. That is where *emotional intimacy* fits in to being a Zen analyst. Zen practice—with its emphasis on whole-hearted and un-self-conscious immersion in whatever we encounter—cultivates this capacity in a psychoanalyst or a psychotherapist.

Psychoanalytic attention to *unconscious communication and meaning*—the second facet of Zen psychoanalysis—enhances the intimacy that meditation fosters. Once I was connected to my psychiatry-maligning teenager, the session-sabotaging client, and the therapist with a severe trauma history, we needed to understand what their words and actions meant.

The third and final aspect of being a Zen analyst is a *special relationship* (and environment) designed to illuminate and transform one's history. Psychoanalysis not only elucidates the interpersonal roots of adult afflictions, but it offers a relationship and experience that is a vehicle for transformation in the present. Central to this kind of relationship is a therapist who is self-reflective, empathic, and creative. The offspring of the union of meditative and psychoanalytic wisdom has the potential to foster remarkable healing and transformation.

References

Freud, Sigmund. *The Interpretation of Dreams*. Standard Edition, 4–5: xxxiii–627. London: Hogarth Press, 1900. (Originally published 1900, pp. 392–393.)

Rubin, Jeffrey B. *A Psychoanalysis for Our Time: Exploring the Blindness of the Seeing I*. New York: New York University Press, 1998.

Rubin, Jeffrey B. "Deepening Psychoanalytic Listening: The Marriage of Buddha and Freud." *American Journal of Psychoanalysis* 69, no. 2 (2009): 93–105.

Rubin, Jeffrey B. *The Art of Flourishing: A New East-West Approach to Staying Sane and Finding Love in an Insane World*. New York: Crown Archetype, 2011.

Rubin, Jeffrey B. *Practicing Meditative Psychotherapy: Pathways to Self-Transformation*. New York: Abiding Change Press, 2013. (Originally published in *The Art of Flourishing: A New East-West Approach to Staying Sane and Finding Love in an Insane World*, 2011, p. 42.).

Suzuki, Daisetz T. *Zen and Japanese Culture*. Princeton: Princeton University Press, 1971.

Vitello, Paul. "Joshu Sasaki, 107, Tainted Zen Master." *New York Times*, August 4, 2014.

Yamada, Koun. "Kyogen's Man Up a Tree." In *The Gateless Gate*, translated by Koun Yamada, 31–34. Tucson, AZ: University of Arizona Press, 1979. (Originally "Mumonkon," 13th century.)

12 The World is Too Much with Us

When Dead Whales, Bigotry, and Vaccinations Join Us in Sessions

In recent years, a new topic has preoccupied psychotherapy patients and therapists alike in an unprecedented way, namely *The World*. Dead whales and school shootings, fake news and authoritarian leaders have entered our offices (or Zoom or Facetime sessions) more intensely and at an ever-quickening pace. To quote William Wordsworth (1807/1948, p. 186), "The world is too much with us."

And this is dividing—and sometimes sabotaging—couples and families, as well as citizens.

"What were you thinking?" a male patient who lives with his wife in the northeast asked her during a couple's session over Zoom. She had just informed him that she was looking for an apartment in Florida.

"That I'd feel more at home there. And that you wouldn't understand because you have been brainwashed by the liberal media," she replied.

"You are deluded," he shot back.

"Right back at ya," she responded.

Their anger was palpable, but so was their hurt and bewilderment. I felt sad, powerless, resourceless. Has anyone healed the antagonisms and alienation people feel in our Age of Rage?

Their destructive vicious cycle of diatribes and devaluations continued until I jumped in.

"In the last five years no one from one side of the massive divide separating Americans seems to have convinced anyone from the other camp about anything," I said. "So, it seems pointless to try."

They remained quiet, but the gulf separating them felt huge—and unbridgeable. They appeared lost in two irreconcilable worlds, not simply opposed political positions.

I was acutely aware of their misery and the insufficiency of my medicine—the talking and listening cure. Had anyone's understanding stemmed the tide of increasing embitterment and fostered reconciliation these last regrettable years?

A movement pattern I practice daily from a Chinese internal martial art called bagua zhang came to mind. I stood up, raised my arms to shoulder

DOI: 10.4324/9781003604730-13

level and stretched my arms sideways with my left palm facing upward and my right hand downward. I visualized ropes pulling my arms in two opposite directions. Next, I elongated my spine and lowered my perineum. And then I tried to stretch in four directions at once without any self-consciousness.

At first, when I practiced what I called four-dimensional stretching, I was mindful of one area—say my left arm—and my right arm would slacken. After more practice, the arms would be stretched, and the upper back or lower waist would loosen. It took practice to be aware of the different facets at the same time. Then I had to be aware of all four dimensions without effort.

After practicing this movement for many months, I said to my teacher: "I feel like Bagua stretches my mind." "My teacher in Taiwan, Luo De Xiu, says 'Bagua expands the mind,'" he replied.

"I believe you love each other," I said to the couple living in contracted universes after I did the Bagua posture. "You are also hurting each other and are certain that the only problem is your deluded spouse. I think you need to shift and broaden your perspective and be a bigger container that holds both of your viewpoints without having to choose between them."

Something shifted in them—they said they felt it, and I could sense it even over Zoom—their diametrically opposed views of vaccinations didn't disappear, but no longer contaminated the love they also felt for each other.

Creating a Bigger Container: Befriending Anger and Fear, Jealousy and Guilt

Cultivating harmony—or at least peaceful co-existence—in the face of contentiousness and agony is easier said than done.

In a culture like our own that is obsessed with feeling happy, challenging emotions—like being angry at our partner—are often indulged or avoided, denied or anesthetized. This harms other people, as well as us.

I cringe when I receive mail about psychological or spiritual workshops on "Getting Beyond Fear" (or Anger). There is no *beyond*, and even if there was it would be harmful to get there because we would be removing vital self-protective and self-healing processes. Fear signals danger and anger often masks disappointment that we need to pay attention to. We don't want to banish that feedback.

Rinzai, a ninth-century Japanese Zen teacher, once said: "Eat when hungry, sleep when tired." I'd add: "Let yourself feel whatever you feel."

When our feelings are greeted by a therapist with empathy and respect it is much easier to accept our experience.

As we create space for our feelings and let them teach us what we care about and are avoiding, an unexpected thing can happen: our anguish can be a bridge to other people. "It was Dostoevsky and Dickens who taught me that the things that tormented me most were the very things that connected me with all the people who were alive, or who had ever been alive," noted James

Baldwin (1963) in an interview with Jane Howard on May 24, 1963, The mad rush in our emotion-averse culture to deny negative feelings and sedate emotional agony robs people of an opportunity to discover what connects us and to broaden our empathy and humanity. And this feels ever more crucial in a world in which parents confront increasing challenges in protecting their innocent children against a world of escalating hate and polarization.

When painful emotions are met with compassion it can grow our heart, expand our circle of concern, and generate lives of greater meaning.

When we can hold our own grief and the sadness of other people more skillfully; we will live and love more wisely.

Creating an oasis of empathy and benevolence and becoming a bigger container for ourselves and in our relationships doesn't eliminate challenging emotions. There is still fear and anger, and all of the other emotions human beings are afflicted by. But we live with them differently—and that may help us bridge seemingly impassable cultural divides about vaccinations, race, or dead whales, or any other emotionally fraught aspect of the world.

References

Baldwin, James. "Doom and Glory of Knowing Who You Are: An Interview with Jane Howard." *LIFE Magazine*, May 24, 1963, 54 (21).

Wordsworth, William. "Sonnet XXIV." In *The Prelude: Selected Poems and Sonnets*, edited by Carlos Baker. New York: Holt, Rinehart, and Winston, 1948. (Originally published 1807.)

13 Escaping the Prison You Didn't Know You Were In

The Covid Jailbreak

Zoom funerals and graduations, financial devastation and pervasive languishing, Covid and its aftermath has been a chronic cultural trauma and an unending nightmare for most people. Sadness and sleeplessness, substance abuse and suicidality are only some of the deleterious consequences.

Covid is the name of a ghastly plague; a reminder of our isolation and alienation; a revealer of how vulnerable we are.

For one client—I'll call him Bruce—the pandemic has also been an unanticipated blessing; a pressure-cooker accelerating unexpected changes and remarkable transformation and healing, rather than imprisonment.

"Dr. R., I just found out my brother has glioblastoma, the brain cancer that felled Ted Kennedy and John McCain," Bruce told me in the fall of 2019.

"The brother you never had is looking at a short-term ticket to the grave," I said. "And I fear that you are in for a wild ride."

"'Life never hands you more than you can handle,' I once heard a Zen teacher say," Bruce responded.

"They have never worked with the torched souls of trauma victims in psychotherapy," I replied.

"I couldn't agree more. Believing that we can and should handle anything is not only excessively idealistic, but also a breeding ground for shame; for blaming oneself when you feel overwhelmed by what Shakespeare called 'the ten thousand natural shocks that flesh is heir to.'"

"How are *you* holding up?" I asked.

"I had an unsettling vision in the middle of the night yesterday."

"Care to share?"

"I am pushed out of a plane. Wind smacks and jerks my body. I feel minuscule in the face of the vast visual expanse that opens up all around me. I am completely disoriented and alone and feel abject terror. I am uncertain of where—and whether—I will land. Or crash. The parachute I didn't know I had opens. I suddenly realize that the plane was a prison and the person who pushed me into free-fall also released me from jail."

"What the hell happened?"

DOI: 10.4324/9781003604730-14

"In the midst of adjusting to my brother's glioblastoma, I just discovered that my partner of 32 years is breaking up with me."

"That we never predicted," I said. "What did she say?"

"I love you. You are my best friend. But I want to live alone. We are on different paths, and you'll be better off without me."

"Two tornados in your life."

" 'Haze sole certitude,' Samuel Beckett wrote in *Ill Seen Ill Said* (1981). I'm shell-shocked. In a daze or haze. And I oscillate."

"Between?"

"Sadness and shame, anger and relief. Sometimes I am lonely and overwhelmed. But now I am nobody's punching bag or scapegoat."

"She was lovely and drove you mad," I said. "You were ambivalent for a long time. She was both a comrade against the annihilating forces of your crazy family, and she inadvertently replicated them and rendered you invisible and voiceless. But that doesn't soften the blow of losing your companion and best friend—the demise of the best home you have ever known."

"The only companion I ever had and thought I could have. Losing her, someone I really trusted, was a cosmic betrayal and threw me back on my primal wound: feeling 'homeless'—that there is no place for me and that I don't belong anywhere."

A Doll's House, Part 3

"It wasn't just *that* she left, Dr. R.," Bruce said to me a few weeks later. "It was *how* she left—the relationship ended without her saying anything. I had to prod it out of her. A 'ghosting' ending—she left without a trace. And that replicated the unimaginably cold and horrifying death of my father several years ago when he exited this life without saying a word to me. I carried around a good deal of anger—intermixed with heavy doses of guilt, fear, and humiliation—for a few weeks until a client of mine, a woman who had blown up her marriage after having an affair, asked me if I had seen *A Doll's House, Part 2*, in which Nora returns to the husband and children she left 15 years earlier."

"I haven't even read the first one," Bruce told her.

"That night I imbibed Ibsen's incendiary play about female enslavement and liberation. And my view of L's behavior—and my fate—radically altered," he added.

"Do tell."

"In the middle of the night I'd remember something she said like 'I am lost, and I don't know what I want or am entitled to' or 'If I don't leave, I'll die' or 'I can't do anything but what I am doing'—and suddenly I would see our relationship from her point of view and get glimpses of what she was striving for and what she hoped to gain, rather than my own hurt or sense of betrayal."

"What do you think she was striving for?"

"I came to feel that she was lost and in torment—not living the life she felt she was meant to live—imprisoned in a world she didn't want to belong to.

Blowing up our relationship may have been a protest against a life that did not feel like her own and a desperate attempt to not lose—and mightily try to find—herself."

"What made her so afraid of losing herself?"

"She was trained since she was 5 to make up for absentee parents and mother her four younger siblings—I remember her telling me years ago that she was standing by a highway when she was 5, alone with her four younger siblings, terrified that one of them would go on the highway and die. She recently said to me: 'Now I don't have to take care of anyone.' I think she organized all of her relationships so that she was a caregiver—who left herself out of the equation—to protect against the dreaded danger she had to face alone as a young child. Even when friends, relatives, and partners fought against this pattern she overrode their efforts, which tragically thrust her back into the depriving experience of childhood. Her 'solution' was a 'prison.'"

"Where are you in all of this?" I asked.

"Lost and floundering. Like a man holding a rope, dangling over an abyss, and losing his grip. I know I won't let go and fall, but I feel like I can't hold on much longer."

The Gift

Bruce shared, "I recently met my friend, Ann, a psychoanalyst, for dinner. She told me, 'A comet has hit your life, Bruce.'"

"How are you doing?" I asked.

"Lonely, lost, and liberated," Bruce replied.

"You don't have to tell me, but it is very important that you know what you are liberated *from*."

"Dr. Rubin, I know the answer and I can tell you. I am liberated from trying to get through to madness . . . Trying to talk to L. about her irrational outbursts, her increasingly contemptuous behavior, trying to get her to see it was not okay to belittle me even if she was hurt or angry."

"My conversation left me with several questions, Dr. R.: 'Why did I settle for madness? Why did I take so much shit? Why did I accept emotional scraps?'"

"You knew no better given your mother's resounding rejection and invalidation of you."

"A nice way of saying: 'You voluntarily agreed to your own debasement.'"

"Or, L. was nicer to you than your mother, but perhaps there is something better out there."

"Which I am clueless about."

"How could you envision what you have never known?"

"That brings to mind a dream I had in high school. I awake and am horrified to find myself in prison. I quickly look around and everyone I know is in prison. We all furiously decorate our cells, which have no locks. As I woke from the dream the following phrase came to mind: 'And they call this living.'"

"What comes to mind about this dream?"

"I used to think it conveyed my belief that most people are caught in the matrix—sleepwalking through their existence. Now I am wondering if the dream also symbolizes what I couldn't then see—my own enslavement. My whole life I have been preoccupied with freedom—probably because I was emotionally incarcerated."

"A prisoner of?"

"Pathological accommodation to other people and diminished expectations. I didn't know what I was entitled to and made do with the scant emotional nourishment that was available. I settled for scraps and that seemed normal, just the way things are. And that's why as an adult I put up with continual verbal attacks and the absence of genuine emotional intimacy with L."

"That's a mouthful—and seems right on target."

"Losing L. is heart-breaking and also liberating. The worst—and best—of times. A tornado that demolishes the familiar and rips away taken-for-granted certainties. You think it might break you, but it leads to an opening, a glimpse of another world that is within this one . . ."

"I want to become an expert in what was shattered and in the world that you are glimpsing."

"I feel freer than I ever have. Not to date and run around—my trust in women is shattered and I am living a monkish existence—but to pursue a life outside of the obliterating confines of my family, with its Eleventh Commandment of 'Thou Shall Not Have a Life.' In the middle of the night a few days ago I wrote the following: 'She freed me from a prison I voluntarily entered. Thanks for the bomb in my living room, which hastened my escape from jail.'"

Sandman No More

"The psychoanalyst D.W. Winnicott somewhere wrote that he became the sand around his patient's feet," Bruce said. "I, too have been a sandman with a well-developed radar for the vulnerability and the needs of the other person, which I then meld around like the sand."

"Such attunement is admirable. And it has a cost."

"Yes. You become an extension of other people, and you lose yourself."

"The well-being of the other person is the Number 1 priority for the sandman, who becomes a 'disappeared,'" I said.

"Sandman is dying," Bruce replied. "I have zero interest in the kind of selfless caregiving that has characterized my life and that leaves me out. It is not healthy for either person."

Freedom and Demons

"But with freedom, Dr. R., came abject terror, which at first I could not comprehend or explain, as I was catapulted into the world of practical affairs—handling septic tank back-ups, financial ledgers, and flooding in the basement—a realm I had always dreaded and avoided and thus never mastered. My long-term exposure to Eastern contemplative and somatic disciplines—meditation and yoga—helped me non-defensively face and become one with my new nightmare: I dove into cooking new recipes and handling home emergencies, and the inevitable challenges that homeowners unfortunately know. Sometimes I was overwhelmed; at other times it was manageable, which was baffling, as well as gratifying."

"What bewildered you?"

"I'm not sure why I dreaded practical stuff; bank statements, water heaters, and sump pumps were not as onerous as I imagined. It's an unsettling case of 'phantom emotional pain.'"

"Phantom emotional pain?"

"You expect to feel emotional agony, but there's nothing present that causes suffering. I was perplexed about my apparently illogical fear until a friend, who is a psychoanalyst, suggested that perhaps part of me is frozen in time—continuing to see and experience the world through traumas from the past—and that's why practical matters have now seemed so arduous. That insight helped me to understand the terror of the unterrifying."

"What was the source—what happened that froze you?"

"The brutalization by my father, a man whose mastery of math was matched by a vicious temper, which he wasn't shy about unleashing on me. My father used to help a neighbor who was home from college with his math homework. In fourth grade I was doing math with him, and I couldn't grasp the material. He began getting mad and screamed at me, which made it more difficult to answer his questions. He got angrier and I began crying and panicking, which led to more screaming and tears and terror."

"A horrendous nightmare."

"One that crippled me for more decades than I care to remember. I realized I linked practical affairs with his emotional brutalization, and I avoided the former to not re-experience the latter. The anticipated pain caused me to shun large swaths of life—from checking whether the car needed oil to consolidating expenses for the accountant. A profound split developed within me between a person who dove into understanding the intricacies of psychotherapy and someone who studiously avoided taking care of the business of everyday life. I not only didn't understand various aspects of concrete existence and was fairly incompetent, I was more interested in reading books, talking with friends, working out or doing nearly anything but fixing leaks, reconciling bank statements, and repairing computers or printers. And I managed to choose partners who were as talented as I was challenged and avoidant. I felt secret shame about the gaps in my knowledge and my difficulty handling these things, but I was greatly relieved that someone else was willing and able to take care of daily life tasks. They enjoyed being competent and were relieved I would handle other emotional and financial aspects of life. Unfortunately, this reinforced being a gifted pseudo-cripple—a competent person who believes and acts like he's incompetent. I was talented at reading people and finding pathways to healing lost souls and terrified about facing the practical minutiae I could not fathom or handle. This system worked—at least for me (actually it didn't even work for me)—until the sudden and unexpected breakup, which thrust me without any preparation into the territory I had organized my life into avoiding. Now it was sink or swim."

"You stayed away from the realm defined and inhabited by your father to avoid re-traumatization."

"Yes. And recognizing the psychology underlying my passivity and avoidance—why I did it and what I gained from that—taught me two other profound things. The first was that pain and constricted living are emotional fire-alarms—signaling what we need to pay attention to rather than tune out—which is a doorway into liberation. They are, in other words, one of the crucial ways to open the unlocked cell in the dream in which we are all imprisoned. Without the impetus emotional conflict and entrapment affords, the forces of the psychological status quo and emotional homeostasis usually leave us incarcerated and paralyzed."

"The partially phobic life that you lived?"

"Yes. The fear and paralysis that have lived within me for decades were breadcrumbs leading me home to the source of the problem. Without the clues they offered I would be enslaved to my terrors and continuing to be a Master of Avoidance."

"What was the other important lesson this nightmare afforded?"

"As I began meditating on the second fear the breakup triggered—never finding an emotional home—I realized that the rootlessness I fear in the future is a profound alienation I experienced in the past as an eternal outsider in my biological family and with my ex. Like in the robot dream."

"You've talked about some of this in the past," I reply, "but it is suddenly hitting me with a massive force. Tell me the dream again."

"I'm in a small room in a basement without a window with my parents. They are robots. Friends of theirs knock on the door. I go to open the door, and I desperately try to nonverbally signal to them with my eyes that something is very wrong. I don't succeed. They come in the room. My parents transform into ordinary-looking people and follow an invisible script floating in the air that only the three of us can see. The dream is terrifying and horrifying."

"That it was—and is. I am haunted by what it was like for you having robots as parents. The horror. The inability to be understood. No one knowing the nightmare you were going through. The loneliness."

"When I first went to therapy as a young adult, I remember saying I had a good childhood. It took me a long time to realize that I was emotionally neglected and abused."

"That you were," I said. "And I need to wake the fuck up so that you are no longer alone against these annihilating forces."

"Covid is a ghastly nightmare," Bruce said. "When I consider the way so many people I know are frightened and shell-shocked, grief-stricken and demoralized, it is unsurprising that they tell me they feel as if they are languishing in jail."

"You don't sound totally convinced," I replied.

"For me the pandemic has also provided an unexpected gift: a chance for both a radical reevaluation of my life and priorities and an opportunity to focus on what really matters."

"A training ground for transformation?"

"Yes," Bruce said. "The quarantine upended my previous existence. Forced to withdraw from my old life, I was more isolated, which generated loneliness. I was also more emotionally immunized against a psychologically crazy world. I cycled through a range of emotions—from dejection and self-pity to clarity and liberation. The opportunity for self-reflection also grew. My solitary existence created an unexpected space in which I was radically thrown back on myself and had the chance to consider what I felt and wanted with minimal impingements."

"Covid was The Great Revealer. You were the marble in Michelangelo's quarry."

"Covid helped me chip away the excess and bring forth the essential."

"Which is?"

"I am awakening from madness—from how absent I was in my own life."

"You are waking up to self-estrangement."

"I realized with greater clarity repetitive patterns and blind spots. Both the quarantine and the time for contemplation became kryptonite for pathological accommodation and sandman. It's as if I woke from a nightmare and a lie—that my life didn't matter. And that my childhood had been stolen. 'Do as I say' and 'believe as I believe' was the silent mandate in my family. All of which led to the crushing weight—and emotional prison—of Bruce-less pathological accommodation."

"How does all of this sit with you *now*?"

"A massive weight has been lifted—and the world feels more like a playground than a foreboding prison cell, although I know there is major work still to be done. I am accommodating less. Speaking up more. Experimenting. Taking risks. I no longer feel like a gifted cripple. Ninjas and air fryers are still a foreign language, but one that I no longer believe is beyond me or I irrationally neglect. Before I was ignorant of practical matters and avoidant; now I am a game newbie."

"Could we say your existence is now authentic—that you are finding and being yourself?"

"Real, alive—and—incomplete."

"Because you are *alone*?"

"Exactly . . . And pessimistic about finding a soulmate."

"And a *home*."

Voyages into the Unknown

"Many people look for 'who they really are,' Dr. R. 'You Be You.'"

"Their 'True Self'?"

"Exactly. They seek a buried blueprint from their past and assume that accessing it will direct and guide them on how to live now."

"The alternative?"

"Self-creation in the present: fashioning who we want to be based on our current values and ideals and the realities and constraints of our existence."

"I am imagining this relates to this new and unfamiliar chapter in your life?"

"I think I have undergone a psychological death to who I thought I was, which creates a void and a possibility."

"You have to be open to the unknown and unexpected."

"Not so easy to envision what I have never experienced."

Going Where He Didn't Want to Go

"Several weeks ago, my friend Diana wrote to me that she didn't understand my pessimism about finding a soul mate."

"What did she say? Why are you blushing?"

"She said I was warm and kind, charming and brilliant. Rare. Diana's comments were a kind of mental chiropractic, which had an unexpected liberating effect and led to a huge breakthrough: it helped me see myself in a new and radically different light, and that snapped me out of my faithlessness. I departed from my contemplative cave, and I immediately joined and wrote a profile for Bumble, which helped me delineate what I was looking for."

"Which is?"

"'My last date, my last love . . . Find out what is worthwhile about yourself and express it,' Linda Lee Cadwell, the widow of Bruce Lee, wisely counsels. The relationship I yearn for is a home for the best of us—a place in which we can each be our most self with the other person—which includes our wisdom and self-blindness, our strengths and vulnerabilities. We would also appreciate the ordinary and extraordinary bounties life has to offer and create a relationship in which we can each stay sane—even sometimes flourish—in a topsy-turvy world."

"This is powerful and unexpected. How is the dating going?"

"Affirming and disorienting, clarifying and demoralizing. I've been dating for a few months and trying to do it in a new way from when I last went out to find a suitable partner some 30-odd years ago—just being myself and seeing if there is a fit, rather than trying to make something happen. I give myself high marks for a good attitude and effort in a scary and mostly unfamiliar world. I feel less on the line—every encounter is not a moratorium on my worthiness—and it is easier to be my real self. It was also heartening to get some positive responses to my Bumble profile, which challenged my entrenched narrative about never finding a partner. And it was exhilarating to reconnect with the playful boy before he was traumatized by his father's brutal reaction to his burgeoning awareness of girls."

"What's been disorienting?"

"The initial positive responses I received to my profile and text exchanges were bolstering—albeit unsettling—because they challenged how I saw myself in relation to women: a quirky, nonconformist with qualities that don't necessarily play well in the dating market, who will always remain a bachelor."

"Did your 'success' challenge your old, familiar, taken-for-granted negative narrative that there's no place for you and that there are only two deadly options: give the other person what they want, surrender your authentic self and have a place, or be yourself and be thrust into isolation and desolation?"

"Absolutely . . . I have begun to wonder if my pessimism is a vision of the world and my prospects within the prison of trauma. Do you think that's why I wrote the other day that I woke up after a date emotionally drunk—like I had emerged from a spin cycle in a dryer?"

"It can be frightening, as well as relieving, to recognize that there just might be a place for you."

"It was."

"You are not convinced?"

"The experience of dating has been ultimately dispiriting. Most of the encounters have been—how can I say it charitably—underwhelming. I have been trapped at dinner with a racist who believed BLM was more toxic than white supremacists; ensnared on a hike with a narcissistic yoga therapist, who was more focused on telling me who they had worked on in the Hamptons than getting to know anything about me. I was, however, mercifully saved from an emotional rollercoaster when a woman who spent the bulk of our first phone conversation complaining about her lonely 90-year-old landlord/neighbor suddenly turned on me and broke off contact. 'You can't love without equality,' a matchmaker I met recently told me. And I didn't feel much equality. Or interest. In fact, I mostly felt left out and discarded as I spent time with excessively self-preoccupied people who acted as if they were the only ones that had a life. I'd rather be home alone."

"How did you get stuck with them?"

"Trust the tale not the teller, D.H. Lawrence recommended. The women I have met on Bumble have consistently misrepresented themselves in three ways: age, appearance, and what my friend, Joan calls the 'brochure copy' that they have written describing themselves. The reality does not match their descriptions or their pictures, which are often ten years earlier. And many of the women have been so focused on not being rejected that they detach before engaging."

"They seem emotionally available, but are not?"

"Yes, or they are available but a hot mess. Like the woman I went out on a date with last weekend who spent the entire evening telling me about her sociopathic ex, who bugged her house and estranged her from her three adult children, one of whom died recently at the ripe old age of 27. Late into the catalog of woe—I mean the date—I asked: 'What do you enjoy doing when you are not thinking about the abysmal horror you have been undergoing?'. . . Of course, her short answer was trumped by a much longer elaboration of her misery . . . I love doing therapy, but I also enjoy being off the clock . . .'"

"Did all of this reinforce the crushing pessimism that you can't find a place that honors what you value?"

"It didn't help. I have been fighting to hold out hope that there might be a possibility of a home I never had. But burned—or wounded—many of the women who contacted me were more focused on finding fatal flaws than getting to know me. It is boring to speak with someone who is hunting for confirmation of a thesis."

"It must have been emotionally demoralizing to free yourself from passive surrender to sadistic domineering—and eschew the crushing weight of living for another person and engaging in unilateral caretaking—only to discover nothingness."

"My challenge is to envision a future that differs from my past—the certain conviction that If I am myself, I'll never find a home."

"I don't know if one can."

"I am creating an authentic life alone. I know I can't fashion a flourishing relationship by myself. And I don't know if that will ever happen. But I can whole-heartedly engage the uncertainty and attempt to build something new. '[T]here is no road'; the poet Antonio Machado wrote (1895/2003), 'you make your own path by walking.' I recognize that I have to contend with old wounds and restrictive convictions and exercise new emotional and relational muscles as I forge this new phase of my life out of the shards of what happened with L. and in my past. Humans have an endless capacity for self-deception, which is why it is crucial to discover the sources of your ignorance, as Bruce Lee recognized. I am trying to use the experience of dating as a mirror to learn about and transform myself—from who I am attracted to, to how I relate to them. 'We tend to pick people who emotionally injure us in ways we are used to,' my friend Gail wisely notes, as some of my ill-fated Bumble encounters sadly illustrated. I also made avoidable mistakes like being seduced by buzz words like 'empathy,' 'compassion,' and 'soulmate,' as well as pictures of attractive women. And I mindlessly accommodated some of these people. The reverse of being too picky is being too undiscerning, ignoring red flags, overriding signals of problems, and settling for emotional scraps, all of which happened as I have bumbled through Bumble. Blinded by good bio copy—and beauty—I landed with a racist and a narcissist. And that's partly on me."

"But a change is afoot. There's a new decisiveness."

"I am waking up to the horror of a stolen childhood and the lie that I don't matter."

"And adulthood."

"What is horrific is not my childhood, which was in certain crucial ways a nightmare, but the fact that I have reached my limit and can't abide by soul murder anymore."

"I can see the manifestations of that disgust and refusal."

"I knew something was changing recently when I didn't respond to the ad of a beautiful women who wanted a highly ambitious and elegant man. Ambition, like most things, is, of course, in the eye of the beholder. I am highly motivated to be there for my son and his kids and my friends; finish several manuscripts; deepen my work with my patients; and master the schools of therapy I am studying, But I am neither elegant nor highly devoted to mortgage my soul to make as much money as possible. I realized that going out with her would be an exercise in trying to get her to yearn for someone fundamentally different than what she claimed she wanted."

"You are spotting the potential mismatches instead of losing yourself in relentlessly trying to get through to them."

"A few years ago my then 9-year-old grand-daughter said to me that if she was a parent of a son who was dating she would tell him to 'Try to get to know the person, see if you like her, can be yourself with her and think about her later.' Armed with her Four Laws of Attraction I'll face the world of dating . . . If truth be told, Dr. R., I secretly hoped that by now there would be a successful outcome and a Hollywood ending: finding my last love and riding off into the sunset."

"Life has an uncanny way of not conforming to our scripted futures."

Bumbling toward a Home

"A follow-up conversation with my friend Diana, the person most responsible for freeing me from my isolative existence during the Covid pandemic, proved unexpectedly illuminating," Bruce said.

"How is it going?" she asked.

"Much ado about nothingness . . . The responses have been dispiriting, but the process for me has been profound. I try to be myself, not force anything, see what is possible. It takes the pressure out of dating and helps me access a buried part of myself—playful, irreverent, authentic."

"You sound so different than last we spoke. Now you sound confident, happy, and at peace; whereas before you were shell-shocked, confused, and pessimistic," Diana said.

"After that phone call, Dr. R., I felt good and later weird. While what Diana said was true, I was also aware of an opposing cross-current that I couldn't quite articulate. At first, I thought it was that I didn't always feel as upbeat as I sounded with Diana. Later, I realized that the issue was deeper. For all my 'Zen dating,' I was still very single. A conversation a few days later with my Zen teacher and friend, clarified what I couldn't quite put into words after I spoke with Diana."

" 'You are nowhere' my [Bruce's] friend said after listening to my account of my conversation with Diana. At first that was deeply troubling, but later it seemed only partially true. I have not yet found a home in this world. I am somewhere, but not yet arrived," Bruce replied.

"As I said last week," Bruce's friend replied, "trying to find a home in this world doesn't interest me."

"We mean two different things," I [Bruce] said. "There's a germ of truth in each of our perspectives. You don't want to be reconciled to an insane world; I need to feel there's a place for me so that I don't drown in alienation."

"What is *home* to you and what exactly bothered you about your conversation with Diana?" I asked.

"Home, for me, is catching up to myself, appreciating my value, feeling at peace with myself, and flourishing with another person. Diana's triumphant narrative hid my confusion, fear, and pessimism."

"Where does this leave you?" I asked. "And what about your conversation with your Zen teacher?"

"The liminal state of no longer being in the contemplative cave and not yet caught up with myself that my friend missed, became clearer in a conversation I had with my friend, John, a week later," Bruce added.

"How's dating going?" John asked.

"Challenging and well."

"People are responding to you—who you are."

"I'm oscillating between comfort with my adult self and feeling like an adolescent. I am accessing an evolving me—the me at work and in my life when I am not with women."

"The emotional side of you is being valued. You're broadening—not just your intellectual side."

"The old, narrower me: the shy, aspiring intellectual was fully me. It was also a compensatory construct. In elementary school I was playful. Then I was beaten down by my father. The imprisoning self-cure—the buttoned-down ideal self—trapped me. The positive responses from women to my playfulness and spontaneity are chipping away at the character armor around the structure designed to protect me from re-traumatization."

"The constructed self was a survival self," John said. "You are becoming free of pathological accommodation. You are becoming unstuck because of your desire and courage to pursue this."

"You need someone who elicits your brilliance, compassion, and humor, as opposed to someone who is too controlling and critical," I said to Bruce.

"I never thought about it that way, Dr. R., although it makes total sense to be with someone who is good to me—and good for me."

"You've been through an extraordinary voyage of discovery before and after Covid. Where does all of this—liberation from The House and demoralization about dating—leave you?" I asked.

"It's not Paradise," Bruce noted, "but I'm out of prison. Perhaps we could call this season of my life: 'The Covid Jailbreak . . . And the first faint intimation of enlightened intimacy.'"

References

Beckett, Samuel. *Ill Seen Ill Said*. New York: Grove, 1981.

Machado, Antonio. "Traveler, Your Footprints." In *There Is No Road*, translated by Mary G. Berg and Dennis Maloney. Buffalo, NY: White Pine Press, 2003. (Originally published 1895.)

Index

For Product Safety Concerns and Information please contact our EU
representative GPSR@taylorandfrancis.com
Taylor & Francis Verlag GmbH, Kaufingerstraße 24, 80331 München, Germany

www.ingramcontent.com/pod-product-compliance
Lightning Source LLC
Chambersburg PA
CBHW070350270326
41926CB00017B/4073